Diet, Shatkarmas
and
Amaroli

–

Yogic Nutrition & Cleansing
for
Health and Spirit

Yogani

From The AYP Enlightenment Series

AYP Publishing

For ordering information go to:

www.advancedyogapractices.com

Library of Congress Control Number: 2007924700

Published simultaneously in:

Nashville, Tennessee, U.S.A.
and
London, England, U.K.

This title is also available in eBook format – ISBN 978-0-9789344-0-8
(For Adobe Reader)

ISBN 978-0-9786496-4-7 (Paperback)

All things in moderation...

Introduction

While the methods of Yoga are many, its underlying principle is very simple. The human body is a doorway between our outer world and a boundless inner realm of peace, love and creative energy. When the doorway has been opened through effective spiritual practices, health, productivity and happiness in daily life are the natural result.

Diet, Shatkarmas and Amaroli provides practical instruction on a range of approaches and techniques that can supplement a daily routine of core yoga practices including deep meditation and spinal breathing pranayama. Once we have begun to cultivate our inner silence, we will naturally be moved to undertake additional means that can enhance our inner purification and opening. The foods we eat and methods we can use for cleansing and rejuvenating the body will naturally receive more attention. Hence, this small volume.

Here we will take a close look at nearly everything we put into our body, as well as what comes out of it, with an eye toward promoting good health, while focusing on time-tested methods for cultivating human spiritual transformation. Happily, the cultivation of both health and spirit are served by the same means.

This is not a *diet book*, not in the way such books are normally thought of – providing specific guidelines on what to eat and not eat according to a fixed ideology designed to fit everyone. Life is not that simple. We all have different needs at different times in our life. This is especially true for those involved in yoga practices, where the inner neurobiology is in constant change toward greater openings. The diet will change accordingly, as will the need for cleansing techniques and other practices. This book is designed to provide useful information on diet and cleansing methods to aid spiritual practitioners in making wise choices on their chosen path.

The AYP Enlightenment Series is an endeavor to present the most effective methods of spiritual practice in a series of easy-to-read books that anyone can use to gain practical results immediately and over the long term. Since its beginnings in 2003, *Advanced Yoga Practices (AYP)* has been an experiment to see just how much can be conveyed in writing, with much more detail provided on practices than in the spiritual writings of the past.

Can books provide us the specific means necessary to tread the path to enlightenment, or do we have to surrender at the feet of a *guru* to find our salvation? Well, clearly we must surrender to something, even if it is to our own innate potential to live a freer and happier life. If we are able to do that, and maintain regular practice, then books like this one can come alive and instruct us in the ways of human spiritual transformation. If the reader is ready and the book is worthy, amazing things can happen.

While one person's name is given as the author of this book, it is actually a distillation of the efforts of thousands of practitioners over thousands of years. This is one person's attempt to simplify and make practical the spiritual methods that many have demonstrated throughout history. All who have gone before have my deepest gratitude, as do the many I am privileged to be in touch with in the present who continue to practice with dedication and good results.

I hope you will find this book to be a useful resource as you travel along your chosen path.

Practice wisely, and enjoy!

Table of Contents

Chapter 1 – You are the City of God

Human beings have remarkable capabilities for achieving what has been called *spiritual experience*. No one is excluded from this possibility. For those who wish to open the inner door, a wondrous world awaits. We don't have to go further than the functioning of our own heart, mind and body. Through these seemingly common aspects of our everyday existence, the infinite can be unfolded from within us. We only need apply some effective methods, or practices.

Thanks to the work of innumerable seekers and sages over thousands of years, there is a wide range of spiritual practices available to us today. Experience has shown that some of these practices are of greater importance than others, mainly because they stimulate fundamental changes within us, which serve as the foundation for subsequent practices and experiences. So there is a logical order of practices that we find can lead us on a logical course of development through the maze of our unfoldment. It is not nearly as difficult as at sounds, assuming we are willing to put the most important practices in place first. From these, everything else will flow more or less automatically.

In the *Advanced Yoga Practices* (AYP) system, we begin with a short, twice-daily routine of *deep meditation*. Within a few weeks or months after learning deep meditation, we can add *spinal breathing pranayama*, which is performed right before our meditation sittings. These two practices constitute the core of the AYP approach. They cultivate two qualities in us that form the foundation for all subsequent practices, and the rise of profound and unending spiritual experience interwoven with our everyday life. Deep meditation cultivates the quality of inner silence, or stillness. Spinal breathing pranayama cultivates the quality of ecstatic conductivity, the flow of divine energy within our body and beyond. With these two aspects of our inner nature rising, a range of other practices can be applied with an effectiveness that will greatly expand our experience. These practices include *samyama, asanas, mudras, bandhas, self inquiry, and tantric sexual methods,* all of which are covered in the AYP writings.

In addition to these practices, some which are quite exotic and formerly esoteric, we also consider the seemingly more mundane aspects of our daily living – what we eat and how we keep our body clean and functioning to best support our health and spiritual development. In the matters of diet and inner cleansing, particular methods can be applied which have been demonstrated to be effective, especially during certain stages of our inner development.

While diet and inner cleansing techniques have most often been thought of in terms of achieving and maintaining good health and longevity, we will take a different angle here. We will view health and longevity as side effects, or the fringe benefits, of sound spiritual practices and progress. Indeed, physical health is a natural outcome from spiritual health.

It has been said that the human body is the *City of God.* For all to be well in the city, it is necessary to begin at the central source with core practices, and then stimulate and regulate the flow of energy throughout the city in a way that will assure growth to the highest level of functioning. Much of this process is automatic, a product of our natural inner evolution. With spiritual methods, we stimulate this natural process. This is how we will consider diet and inner cleansing methods.

A Branch of Yoga called "Purity"

Yoga is one of the most comprehensive systems of spiritual practice that has been handed down to us over the centuries. Yoga means "union," or "to join." The methods of yoga facilitate the union, or joining, of our inner and outer nature, the joining of the divine and worldly aspects of us. This is why we often refer to the human nervous system as the doorway between this world and the divine. All we have to do is open the door, and we can live a divine life here on earth. There is no need to go away to the mountain top. No need to quit our job, give away our possessions, or leave our family. As we apply the methods of yoga for a few minutes each day, we can go on just as before, only being much happier and effective in our daily life. This is the real benefit of yoga.

The traditional system of yoga is described in the *Yoga Sutras of Patanjali*, and consists of eight limbs:

- **Yama** (restraints)
- **Niyama** (observances)
- **Asana** (postures)
- **Pranayama** (breathing techniques)
- **Pratyahara** (introversion of the senses)
- **Dharana** (attention on an object)
- **Dhyana** (meditation – dissolving the object)
- **Samadhi** (absorption in pure consciousness)

The combined use of the last three limbs of yoga with a particular technique called *samyama* yields what we call *stillness in action* in daily living.

The first two limbs of yoga, *yama (restraints) and niyama (observances)*, constitute what we call the *codes of conduct*. It is similar to what we find in all of the spiritual traditions of the world – "don't do this," "do this," etc.

The restraints and observances include:

- **Yama** (restraints) – ahimsa (non-violence), satya (truthfulness), asteya (non-stealing), brahmacharya (preservation and cultivation of sexual energy) and aparigraha (non-covetousness).

- **Niyama** (observances) – saucha (purity), samtosa (contentment), tapas (heat/focus/austerity), svadhyaya (study of spiritual writings and self) and isvara pranidhana (surrender to the divine).

Note that *saucha* (purity) is the first observance. This is where we find the principles of diet and shatkarmas (bodily cleansing techniques). Saucha is the branch of yoga that deals with the aspects of conduct that receive a lot of attention in our modern world. Many of us live in a culture that is obsessed with diet and the physical body. In yoga, saucha is important. Yet it is but one branch in the broad spectrum of our practices.

While many traditional approaches to teaching yoga regard yama (restraints) and niyama (observances) as prerequisites for beginning practices further down the list of the eight limbs, some other teachings (including AYP) do not take this view. Yama and niyama can also be regarded as effects in an integrated approach to engaging in practices, beginning with deep meditation, pranayama, postures and other methods, irrespective of our adherence (or not) to the conduct guidelines of yama and niyama.

<u>When an integrated approach to practices is taken, yama and niyama are found to be arising naturally as effects.</u>

This occurs through a quality within everyone that we call the *connectedness of yoga*. In other words, one practice used as *cause* will beget other practices as *effect*. The deeper the practice we use as cause, the more profoundly will additional limbs of yoga be stimulated. And so it goes.

If we begin with deep meditation and spinal breathing pranayama as core practices, then we will find aspects of practice contained within yama and niyama rising naturally as effects. These effects will then add further causes to our practice routine, much more so than if we had taken on the methods of yama and niyama alone at the beginning.

This has great significance when considering diet and inner cleansing methods. If we utilize the yogic principles of diet and cleansing methods as a result of rising inner silence and ecstatic conductivity cultivated within us via deep meditation and spinal breathing pranayama, we stand to gain much more. On the other hand, if we force the issue of conduct by blindly adhering to external rules, we can create more obstacles to our spiritual progress than we will remove, in the form of forced behaviors and increasing self-judgment. If our conduct in matters of diet and inner cleansing methods is coming naturally from within, rather than enforced from outside, then we stand to gain much more from the measures presented in this book.

A wise approach to engaging in the practices here is to become grounded in the core practices of deep meditation and spinal breathing pranayama first. Then the principles of saucha (purity and cleanliness) will be rising from within us naturally.

In the AYP approach to practices, we devote selective attention to yama and niyama, as necessary, to support a quick start in deep meditation, spinal breathing pranayama and other practices. Then the yamas and niyamas will be greatly boosted by these powerful practices and will blossom naturally.

Does this mean we do not concern ourselves with diet at all in our life? Of course not. What it means is that we cannot find health or happiness through forced conduct. The best approach is to avoid extremes and take all things in moderation, *favoring* the measures we know will bring us greater health and happiness. Over time, our path will become more clear, and we can let our conduct in these matters shift gradually according to our intuition, which will be steadily rising with our inner silence and ecstatic conductivity, as we continue with our yoga practices.

Along the way, our inner perception will become very refined, and we will learn to listen to our body and follow its lead in many things, including diet and inner cleansing. At some point, we may also find ourselves naturally considering the controversial practice of *amaroli* (urine therapy), a powerful rejuvenation technique, which relates to both diet and inner cleansing.

Nine Gates of the Body

In the ancient lore of yoga, the *City of God* analogy is taken a step further. The City is said to have *nine gates*. These are the natural orifices of the human body, which include two eyes, two nostrils, two ears, the mouth, the urethra and the anus. To take both genders fully into account, which they did not do very well in the old days, we should mention that a woman has ten gates (adding the vagina). It will not make much of a difference in the methods described in this book, though it does in other areas of yoga, particularly *tantra*.

Here, we are concerned with the nourishment of the body and with cultivating the inner energies. On the physical level, it is about what goes in and what comes out. On a more subtle level it is about supporting purification and opening in the subtlest strata of our neurobiology. We will look at eating that way – *diet*. We will look at the cleansing techniques that way – *shatkarmas*. And we will also look at the recycling of urine in the body that way – *amaroli*. All of it is aimed at supporting what we call the rise of *ecstatic conductivity* in the nervous system. As such, the practices will be to support specific neurobiological connections, including:

- **Mouth, Urethra and Anus** – in relation to the neurobiology of the gastrointestinal (GI) tract.

- **Nasal Passages, Eyes and Ears** – in relation to the neurobiology of the brain and spinal nerve.

By influencing the flow of energy and/or nourishment through these gates, we can greatly assist the rise of ecstatic conductivity throughout the entire nervous system.

These measures, along with the rest of the practices covered in the *AYP Enlightenment Series*, will aid the continuing expansion of inner silence and ecstatic conductivity, leading to refinement of all of our sensory perceptions and experiences. It will happen as we engage in the practices of diet, shatkarmas and amaroli in a natural way, when we are called to them from within.

The Call from Within

What is it that moves us to make a change in our diet, or to undertake a yoga practice that we might have considered to be a bit strange before? Why change anything in our living habits at all?

The most common reasons why we make such changes is because of how we feel. In other words, it is for our health and wellbeing that we are most often moved to make changes in our diet and other aspects of our routine. It is cause and effect.

If we are overweight and feel poorly, one the first things we will do is try and find the will to lose some weight. A multi-billion dollar industry has grown up around this simple urge to feel better. In addition, we might not feel so good because our body lacks physical exercise. When the body sags, so do the mind and the emotions. So, another multi-billion dollar industry has grown up around physical exercise.

All we would like is to feel better, to feel whole!

And what does it mean to feel whole? Obviously, if we take it on the physical level only, it means to be healthy and in good physical condition – diet and exercise.

Yet, someday we will get old. No matter how well we eat or how much we exercise, we will eventually be fading away physically. That is life on this earth. We are born, we live for however long our time allows, and we die. Is that all there is? If so, there is no need to read further, because a healthy lifestyle alone will be enough to achieve our fifty or one hundred years, and there are plenty of places we can find advice in those multi-billion dollar diet and exercise industries. How much more are we willing to do to gain a few more years on this earth?

Or maybe just feeling better today is enough. If that is our goal, then this opens up a new avenue, because it is possible to *always* feel good today, even as the body is fading away in old age or other maladies that will claim our body sooner or later. It is possible for us to always feel okay, no matter what the external circumstances may be. This is a spiritual attainment. It is *something more* that reaches far beyond what the diet and exercise industries can deliver. Enter the yoga industry – not nearly as large, but growing, while overlapping diet and exercise and adding a whole new dimension, a spiritual dimension.

In yoga, we recognize the basics of healthy living, and there is much more we can do as well. The methods of yoga can not only add to our longevity, but also look far beyond the limitations of our physical body to our spiritual dimensions.

We each have natural abilities within us that can be stimulated through various methods to unfold a greater potential. This potential is outside time and the ups and downs of our body and everyday living.

Yet these qualities can be cultivated while we are living a normal life, and can sustain us through all of our life experiences – "in sickness and in health."

If we are able to consciously become that which is permanent happiness within us, then what happens to the body will not bowl us over. Inner silence and ecstatic radiance are the qualities we are speaking of here. With those qualities becoming our full time experience in life, we have solved the *feeling good* question for all of this life, and beyond.

We can call it *enlightenment*.

Deep inside each of us is a recognition of our possibilities, and at times we will feel the pull. Actually, we feel it all the time. It is our longing for more happiness in all of its forms. So our desire to feel better is a call coming from within.

If we are engaged in yoga practices like deep meditation, spinal breathing pranayama, and others, the call coming from within us refines. Our sensitivities refine along with our urges, and we are called to do those things we did not even imagine before. We might question our own inner urges. Yet, with yoga practices in the picture, we will gradually learn to trust the call coming from within. We will learn to trust our refining intuition.

If we keep up yoga practices over the long term, the decision-making for healthful living gets easier – obvious even. Not that we know the outcome of all things, or that it will always seem to be what we want. We come to know that inner silence is the best launching pad for all outcomes in our life. Our inner silence emanates a knowing beyond understanding. Experience bears this out over time. This is how abiding inner silence gained in deep meditation fulfills the conditions of yama and niyama.

But more than that, we become our own compass

at the deepest level of spiritual unfoldment, which is beyond the rules of yama and niyama. It is freedom to choose in a way that is life supporting for ourselves and for all who are around us.

Chapter 2 – Yogic Diet

The subject of human diet is a vast and diverse field, filled with experts having impeccable credentials, with many taking opposing views about what we should be eating and not eating. The endless debates on diet can be very passionate, and often become tangled and confused. We will try not to take sides.

Actually, the minute details of diet will be dealt with fairly lightly here, in a way that encapsulates the essentials from the point of view of a fully integrated approach to yoga practices. If we can understand our relationship to diet well enough to allow a natural evolution of our eating habits in concert with the call of our rising inner silence, then the rest will take care of itself.

Here, we will take a closer look at how diet relates to spiritual growth, and in so doing, we will naturally ferret out the essentials of healthy eating. It is not so complicated if we are working from our center, rather than attempting to judge all the details. This is the key to considering diet on the spiritual path. After all, if our body is telling us what we should be eating for our health and spiritual well-being, and we have developed the ability to listen and favor those natural inner tendencies, then what more needs to be said?

Are We What We Eat?

There is the old saying, "You are what you eat." We are going to take exception to that statement. It only applies if we believe we are our body, and that takes who we really are out of the equation. It is just food and the body. So, who is eating?

The primary reason why nearly all diet plans fail beyond the first few months is because these plans are body-based, and do not take into account who it is that is behind the eating. They presume that we are what we eat.

The truth of the matter is that we are not what we eat. We are *unbounded pure bliss consciousness*, and nothing that happens on this earth plane can change that reality.

We only need realize what we are, even as we are living in this body here and now. As we do, our life will gradually evolve to reflect the *truth* that lives eternally within us, which is us. Our eating habits will evolve along with the refinement in our perceptions and actions in every part of our life. If this sounds simple, it is!

Ask anyone who has been practicing deep meditation for a few weeks or months, and you will be likely to hear that, along an increasing awareness about how to improve happiness through conduct in everyday living, there is also an increase in awareness about healthy eating. It just happens.

What is healthy eating?

This is a question often asked by those who are becoming more aware of what they are putting in their body.

"What can I do to improve my eating?"

The question may not even be associated with weight or health concerns. It is simply a question on how to express inner values better in daily living. Diet motivation coming in this way is not based mainly on material concerns. Because it is coming primarily from within, rather than being body-based, it will have a timelessness associated with it. This is the kind of diet motivation that will have staying power and yield lasting results. It is change that does not rely only on the force of will (which sooner or later will fail), but on the force of *truth* radiating from within us.

With the question coming from the right place deep within us, we automatically know what is right action. Then the specific information about what to eat is practically an afterthought, because right conduct is inevitable once the call from within is being clearly heard. Then any information that is given will ultimately lead to the right place.

For those who are engaged in yoga practices, and feeling the call for more harmonious eating coming from within, we can offer some general guidelines.

In the AYP writings, we have previously boiled it down to one phrase – allow your eating to evolve naturally toward *light and nutritious*.

Light and nutritious is synonymous with the Sanskrit/English term *sattvic diet*, which means *yogic diet*.

Believe it or not, this is all the advice a dedicated yoga practitioner needs, and even that may not be necessary, with the inner guidance leading to purification and opening that is readily available to all who are engaged in deep meditation and other yoga practices on a daily basis. Nevertheless, we will go further and expand on that basic advice here, looking at the key aspects of diet from a yogic point of view.

Diet and Health

While it is true that healthy eating is an important factor in creating and supporting good health, we still regard diet to be an intermediary step between who we are (pure bliss consciousness) and how we are manifesting our inner essence physically on this earth. By going beyond diet with yoga practices, we will find our essential motivation for becoming all that we can be in this life.

Interestingly, we will often come to this spiritual realization when faced with the hard facts of our physical existence – our health and our mortality. It is these factors that drive us toward that mystical *something more* that we are all seeking in life. For many of us, the spiritual quest begins and continues with a quest for physical health. We have to start somewhere, and it is the obvious place to take a stand. However, diet is not where our quest for health and happiness should end. If it does, we have missed something important, not the least of which is the primary motivation for healthy living, which has its genesis within us, not outside us.

However we have come to consider diet, our actions will reflect our own *style*. Our choices will incorporate whatever information we have encountered in the vast marketplace of diet systems, our personal preferences, the influence of our role models, and even our sense of morality about what we eat.

Our ancient ancestors ate what was available in whatever location they happened to be living, with little control over the outcome. If the soil was good and the weather suitable, combined with good accumulated agriculture skills, then the people thrived. On the other hand, if conditions were poor, the society fared accordingly. The birth and rise of human civilization (including all technology) can be traced back to the fertile locations on the earth.

Nowadays, the challenge of diet and nutrition has been turned completely on its head. In many parts of the world, it is *choice* that determines what we eat, more than the dictates of a limited selection. This is not true everywhere, of course, but for most who may be reading this book, dietary choice is part of the equation. So, rather than being dependent on the elements, most of us are dependent on our ability to choose wisely and eat in moderation. If we don't do either, we will be prone to suffer ailments that can rival the problem of not having enough food of any kind!

Weight Loss

In western societies there is a huge focus on body weight, for both vanity and health reasons. It is well known that excess body weight is related to a litany of health issues, and can substantially shorten our life, by decades in some cases. This is not to pass judgment on body weight, or even on what a person's body weight is supposed to be. The length of life is not the primary measure of happiness. Happiness is always in the now, and not much related to a person's body weight. Yet, longevity is related to body weight, so if we are seeking longevity, along with our happiness, some attention on diet will be appropriate.

There are many approaches to weight loss. In all cases, the formula is to eat less on a regular daily basis. In fact, the simplest diet one could imagine can be summed up as, *consistently eat less*.

There are a thousand strategies for doing this, ranging from fasting to eating large quantities of low calorie foods. And in recent years, strategies have emerged involving eating less of foods that stimulate the body to store fat, and more of foods that do not stimulate the body to store fat – the so-called low carbohydrate, high protein and fat diets. This is in contrast to the lower fat, higher carbohydrate diets that have been in favor over the past few decades.

Whether one is from the low carbohydrate camp or from the low fat camp, one underlying truth prevails – fresh fruits, vegetables, foods with good fiber content, and adequate water consumption will be important parts of any diet. This has been demonstrated time and time again, whether we are considering diet from the standpoint of weight loss or improving health. It is also true that processed foods that artificially increase carbohydrate and/or fat content and include chemical additives will not necessarily be a positive component of any diet.

But what of the low carbohydrate versus low fat debate?

There is nothing to debate, really, because both are right as long as they are taken in moderation. Too much carbohydrate (sugars and starches) in the diet is not healthy. Too much fat (animal or vegetable) in the diet is not healthy either, particularly saturated fat. By the same token, a zero carbohydrate diet is extremely unhealthy, just as a zero fat diet is extremely unhealthy.

The benefits of both can be gained by eating both natural carbohydrates and fats in moderation.

In fact, the issue of weight loss is taken care of automatically if one moves toward a balanced diet including a variety of fruits and vegetables, moderate amounts of carbohydrates (mostly from fruits, vegetables and whole grains), and modest amounts of protein and fats, along with adequate water consumption and foods with good fiber content. Moderate use of nuts, herbs and spices can add significant nutritional value as well.

Losing weight is about eating less on a regular basis. That means at all our regular meal times, not only now and then, or on a reverse binge basis. Drastic reductions in food intake, or an obsession with not eating (anorexia) can be as unhealthy as eating too much all the time. Balance is the key.

Good eating habits cannot be regimented from outside. No diet system will work long term if the call is not coming from within on an ongoing basis. This is why daily deep meditation may be the single best diet measure anyone can undertake. As inner silence comes up, our conduct automatically shifts to more healthful balanced living, which is a natural component of yoga.

Overcoming Hunger

In the context of this discussion, *hunger* does not mean what is experienced by those who are living in poverty and do not have enough to eat – far too many people around the world. The solution for that kind of hunger is to provide food, plus the means to eliminate poverty and the ill that it breeds.

Most who are reading here will not be suffering from real hunger. Rather, what we call *hunger* in modern society is a conditioned response in the body to a reduction in food consumption from what we have been accustomed to. Chances are, what we have been accustomed to eating is more than is necessary to nourish the body and maintain good health, sometimes giving us the opposite effect instead – declining health. Behind excessive food intake are the hunger pangs that can come upon us a few hours, or even a few minutes, after we have eaten a meal.

What is this hunger that drives us to excessive eating, and how do we overcome it?

While there is some evidence that genetics are involved in overeating and obesity, such cases represent a small minority. Much of the rest of society has simply slipped into the habit of unhealthy eating. The food industry, ever mindful of its bottom line, hasn't been helpful in this regard, heavily promoting foods that are ever more pleasing to the palate, and chemically addictive besides. These are the foods loaded with processed carbohydrates, sugars and fats. These are the very foods that can leave us feeling a deficit, and hungry soon after consuming them, even if we are bloated. The effects of these foods on the digestive processes and blood sugar produce a roller coaster in our neurobiology, plus strong tendencies toward weight gain, diabetes, cardiovascular disease, and many other ailments.

Yet, the hunger pangs keep us coming back to these foods, which are readily available on practically every street corner. It is most risky for those whose career or lifestyle require eating out in restaurants often.

Regardless of the culture we live in, what we have been eating, and where we are eating, we do have the last word on what goes into our body. It is our choice. If we understand that what we are dealing with is our own habit, then we will also know that the habit can be changed, reprogrammed for better health and spiritual growth.

The call must come from within. There is no one who can reprogram our conduct the way our own inner wisdom can. This is why deep meditation and other spiritual practices form the first line of strategy. As we purify and open the inner neurobiology, the desire and will to engage in healthier eating habits will be there. As we cultivate more inner silence, we will be able to see our hunger for what it is – a biochemical reflex. We will be able to experience it with less compulsion to act upon it. In time, we will come to know that our hunger is actually a call for purification. As we allow ourselves to be with it without acting, we will come to know that behind this hunger is great power for purification. As we continue to allow it without acting, we can feel our inner energies shifting away from the habitual anticipation of digestion and blood chemistry imbalance toward the much broader agenda of inner purification. Hunger then becomes a positive symptom of inner purification, and we can enjoy it, because we know it is regenerative.

When we do eat, we will be inspired to shift toward more balance in our diet, and away from processed foods that artificially stimulate the hunger habit.

All of this comes from cultivating more inner silence in deep meditation. Additional help can be found for overcoming hunger with *samyama*, a practice that enables us to move our inner silence for particular effects. Also, as inner silence continues to rise, we may be inspired to explore *fasting* (below) and other methods that can enhance our health and spiritual progress.

Whatever our eating habits have been in the past, we do have the power within us to change them. As we find our center in stillness we will come to know that our hunger is only a habit, a reflex, and that we can utilize it as a stimulus for purification and opening leading ultimately to a dramatic reduction of its hold over us.

Overcoming hunger is one aspect of our journey of inner discovery, leading to better health and increasing happiness in all aspects of life.

The Road to Cardiovascular Health

High blood pressure, coronary disease, heart attacks and strokes have been epidemic in western societies, and have been gradually spreading to the eastern societies as western eating habits and lifestyles have.

The good news is that awareness has been steadily rising in the west over the past few decades, and the cause and effect relationship between diet/lifestyle and cardiovascular health has become clear. The result has been the rise of the vast diet and exercise industries, and increasing pressure on the old habits of smoking and excessive alcohol consumption, which are also major contributors to disease.

It should not be surprising that the formula for good cardiovascular health is not very different from the formula for weight loss, with fine-tuning to round out the health equation. While simply eating less on an ongoing basis will lead to weight loss (at least for a while), overall cardiovascular health requires the following:

- A balanced diet containing a variety of fruits and vegetables, favoring reduced fat and salt consumption.

- Regular aerobic exercise – the equivalent of 20 minutes or more of brisk walking at least four times per week.

- A balanced routine of regular daily activity and rest. Not too much activity, not too much rest.

There is nothing esoteric in these suggestions. For those who suffer cardiovascular challenges, the solutions are straight forward, coming from both modern medicine and ancient yogic advice.

Daily aerobic exercise is one of the first prescriptions to build a healthier cardiovascular system. Whether it be high blood pressure, or other cardiovascular issues, daily exercise and a low fat, low salt, vegetarian diet are good for both the heart and the blood pressure.

Of course, for those with cardiovascular issues, any exercise program should be undertaken in consultation with a doctor.

A yoga friendly exercise program can be found in the *AYP Easy Lessons for Ecstatic Living* book and the smaller *Asanas, Mudras and Bandhas* book.

Interestingly, it is not unusual for some of the traditional yogic diets to have a lot of fat and salt in them, so eating a traditional yogic diet alone may not be adequate to support good cardiovascular health. The addition of modern knowledge is advised, so we have a blend of the old and the new. Both ancient and modern systems have much to offer, and an integration of sound principles from both will yield the best results.

Changing our eating habits and exercise priorities for the good will also change the way we carry on our daily routine, including the work schedule we keep and our relationships with other people. Putting some emphasis on our physical health will affect our life in nonphysical ways, reducing the stress in our life, which is good for our health also.

Some *letting go* is necessary to make these simple but life-altering changes, and that can reduce contractions within our cardiovascular system, and in our heart especially. An opening heart is one that knows how to let go. An opening heart also knows how to laugh!

Of course, all of this is much easier to undertake if we are already engaged in an integrated system of yoga practices. Then we receive a lot of support coming from our inner silence, where all health originates.

Must We Become Vegetarians?

Is it necessary to become a strict vegetarian to achieve good health, and be suitably prepared for yoga practices such as deep meditation?

No, it isn't. All of the suggestions given above can be acted upon within a diet regimen that includes meat and dairy products. It is only a matter of eating in moderation, and favoring the basic guidelines as best we can without throwing our personal preferences out the window. There is no black or white in this. While it seems to be human nature to believe it is so, few things in life *are all or nothing.* So, good health can certainly be maintained by eating a wide range of foods in moderation. For those who have an aversion to fresh fruits and vegetables, try compromising and eating some of these – only a little bit on a regular basis. It won't kill you. If you are a heavy meat eater, favor eating less meat, and see how much better you feel. It can be as simple as favoring lighter meats (like fish or fowl) over heavier meats. These tendencies will come up by themselves if you are practicing deep meditation. It happens like that. Nothing is all or nothing. We just favor what we know will be good for our health and well being. It is logical, yes?

On the spiritual side it is just the same. We eat according to our preferences, favoring what we know will improve our health and well being. A vegetarian diet may gradually emerge in our life as we move ahead, but only if we are naturally inclined that way.

Forced diets are not the best diets, because they introduce stress and self-judgement. The first chance it gets, the body rushes back to the old diet. This is why regimented diet programs rarely work over the long run. It has to come from within. The same goes for morality-based diets – avoiding certain foods for moral reasons. Our rising spiritual instincts will guide us more harmoniously than rules of conduct or rigid ideologies imposed externally.

If we are meditating regularly, we will find that, in time, we will be drawn to a lighter, more nutritious diet. Our preferences will change naturally. And we can trust that. The body knows what it needs to sustain the process of purification fostered by deep meditation. As inner silence (pure bliss consciousness) rises, our eating habits will change accordingly.

If it is our choice, it is possible to fulfill all of our dietary needs in a pure vegetarian (vegan) diet, providing for complete protein needs through the blending of seeds, nuts and legumes. It is also possible to fulfill our dietary needs in a healthy way eating a non-vegetarian diet. There are no absolutes in this – only the honoring of personal preferences, and favoring moderation in all things.

Light and nutritious says it all. *Light* to aid in easy cleansing of the nervous system through our yoga practices, and *nutritious* to support good health of the body. Too light is not usually nutritious, and too nutritious is not usually light. Balance is the key. Regular deep meditation will naturally lead us in that direction. A preoccupation with diet is not an aid to meditation, or to anything else in life. So we take it easy and meditate twice each day. If we do that, the diet will take care of itself.

Vitamins, Herbs and Supplements

If we are eating a balanced diet with a good assortment of fruits and vegetables, all of our nutritional needs will be taken care of. If we cultivate good dietary habits, there will be no need for supplemental vitamins and minerals. If the diet is not

so good, then supplements can serve a need, thoug̶
they cannot fully compensate for imbalances in the
diet.

Dietary supplements of all kinds are taken by
hundreds of millions of people around the world
every day. It is another one of those multi-billion
dollar industries that has grown out of our concerns
about diet and health. If the diet is already good,
taking supplements may be regarded to be *insurance*,
just in case our diet has a few nutritional holes in it.
And if the diet is poor, the supplements may serve a
much larger perceived role. The truth is, all the pills
in the world are not going to compensate for a poor
diet. In that case, taking supplements is a misguided
strategy that masks the real issue. It is not about the
nutrients we are not receiving in our diet. It is about
all the things we are putting in that are detrimental to
our health. If we step back behind the behaviors, we
may find that the supplements are being used to avoid
a more fundamental issue that is transcending dietary
considerations.

Why is it that we take supplements? No doubt we
all swear by one or two, at least, convinced that we
have found the way to avoid the common cold, or
have secured the proverbial fountain of youth in a
magic pill. Maybe so, but a good daily routine of
yoga practices leading to a balanced diet and lifestyle
will do much more for our health and longevity than
dietary supplements ever can.

It is okay to take supplements, as long as we are
realistic about their use in relation to the rest of what
we are doing in our life. There is no single magic
bullet that will give us good health. And there is no
handful of pills every morning that can do it for us
either. However, there is magic in developing a
balanced overall approach to living from the inside
out. Lasting happiness can be found by going to our
silent center within, and then learning to act from

they say, happiness cannot be found in a
~~ ~cluding in a pill bottle.

~~~ould be mentioned that the herbal medicine
~~~us of China, India and the indigenous native
~~~res of the world are highly developed, with
ce..turies of accumulated knowledge. The application
of these natural medicine systems is based on specific
causes and effects for the prevention of specific
diseases, or their cure, developed over thousands of
years. It is a specialized area of knowledge that does
not lend itself to casual experimentation like we see
happening so often in the field of dietary
supplements, sometimes with more risk than is
anticipated.

There are benefits that can be gained by
consulting with or studying the work of experts in the
application of herbal preparations. What is there in
the ancient health systems is valuable and can
complement the considerable capabilities of modern
medicine, and, in some cases, delay or eliminate the
need for more radical medical measures. In fact, our
modern pharmaceutical industry utilizes substances
found in the ancient healing systems far more than is
generally known.

Of course, the best insurance against disease is a
lifestyle that promotes good health and the prevention
of mishaps. This is where the spiritual aspect of our
life plays an essential role.

Diet, Spiritual Development and Kundalini

It should come as no surprise that a diet that is
good for our health is also one that that can be an aid
to our spiritual progress – *light and nutritious*.

Can diet be a primary spiritual practice? While
some believe that all things can be solved with diet,
and go to great lengths to make it so with some
extreme behaviors of eating or non-eating, we have to
be realistic and say that diet is an aid to spiritual
development, not a primary cause. If it were a

primary means, the ancient *Yoga Sutras* would surely have diet as one of the major limbs, and we would have many more enlightened diet enthusiasts running around. In the *Yoga Sutras*, diet is, in fact, in the sub-limb of *purity* under the niyamas (observances). In other words, we can't likely eat (or fast) our way to enlightenment, but we can help things along considerably with diet if we are doing more powerful spiritual practices like deep meditation, spinal breathing pranayama, asanas, mudra, bandhas, etc. Then, diet can add another layer of purification and opening to enhance the effectiveness of other practices and our overall progress.

It is often reported by those who are doing deep meditation and other spiritual practices, that diet preferences shift naturally over time – *the call from within*. As our consciousness rises, so will our awareness of healthy eating, as well as a natural urge to do so. And if we don't feel the urge? Well then, let's not worry about it too much. All things in their own time. Taking a forced approach to diet and lifestyle issues will not provide for lasting results. It is pretty certain that a forced diet will be a failed diet in the long run. So, work it from within with sound spiritual practices, and the external habits will follow in time.

"Seek first the kingdom of heaven, and all will be added to you."

Diet and the Neurobiology of Kundalini

As we engage in our spiritual practices over months and years, we are gradually coaxing our nervous system to move to a higher level of functioning. Many of the characteristics of this are measurable in our neurobiology. And quite a few of the changes that are occurring are directly observable. A complex process of purification and opening is occurring in those who practice yogic methods.

There are two main aspects to our purification and opening, each with its own biological signature.

- The Rise of *Inner Silence* – an abiding inner quietness, or stillness, that is beyond our thoughts, feelings and the ups and downs of daily life. We come to know this as our "self."

- The Rise of *Ecstatic Conductivity* (Kundalini) in the Body – sensations of pleasurable energy moving within us, penetrating every aspect of our neurobiological functioning. We come to know this as the "radiant aspect of our self."

While diet is not a primary cause of these changes in our inner functioning, it is a participant in them.

As we find more abiding stillness within ourselves coming with daily deep meditation, we will naturally be drawn to a lighter more nutritious diet.

Likewise, as the neurobiological changes associated with a stirring kundalini begin to occur within us, our diet preferences may change. In addition, certain diet adjustments may be helpful to aid us in navigating some of the excessive energy symptoms that can occur as our inner experiences advance. The process of kundalini is famous for its many symptoms, which can include sensations of heat or coolness in the body, surging emotions, physical vibrations or bodily movements, visions, occasional dizziness or nausea, etc. Sometimes there can be some pain as inner energy (prana) is moving through areas where there are remaining obstructions in our nervous system. All of these symptoms eventually give way to much higher and enjoyable experiences.

Depending on the pattern of inner obstructions in our nervous system and the degree of prudence we exercise in *self-pacing* our practices, we may experience little in the way of uncomfortable symptoms – just steadily increasing ecstasy and bliss, which can bring its own challenges (distractions from stable practice). Regardless, when kundalini becomes active, a good knowledge of yoga practices and the methods of regulating them will pay off in a big way. For those who experience an unmanaged kundalini awakening without knowledge of the particulars involved, it can be a challenging experience, lasting sometimes for years.

Once the kundalini process has begun within us, it can be managed by *self-pacing* our practices in ways that maintain good progress with reasonable comfort. It is a long term transformation we are engaged in, leading to a permanent condition of abiding inner silence, ecstatic bliss, and divine love radiating naturally outward from within us in all that we do in daily life.

Digestion is at the center of the kundalini process and many of its associated symptoms. So it stands to reason that diet has a role to play. And the role of diet will not always be the same, depending where we are on our path. To understand this better, let's look at the process occurring in the gastrointestinal (GI) tract in a person who has an active kundalini, and how this relates to diet.

While there are many aspects to the functioning of kundalini, both physical and non-physical, we will focus on the physical here, as far as we can go with it. For the purpose of this discussion, we will take the view that spiritual experience rises from neurobiological processes occurring in our body. There are more mystical ways of looking at it, and there is nothing wrong with that. It is the same process occurring, no matter how we choose to describe it. When we are reviewing the effects of diet (and shatkarmas and amaroli in the next two chapters) looking at the biology can be helpful, as far as we can trace it with direct perception. There is little doubt that modern science will be taking a much closer look at the neurobiology of kundalini in the years and decades to come. It is the next great frontier of scientific exploration – the causes and effects of human spiritual transformation!

Kundalini is traditionally viewed as the *awakening* of a vast latent energy located near the base of the spine, which rises up the spine to the head. There, a union occurs between the rising energy and stillness, with the energy being feminine (shakti) and the stillness being masculine (shiva).

When we look at the experiential neurobiology of this, a few more components can be added, which are consistent with the metaphors found in many of the world's scriptures, including the more direct descriptions found in Indian Yoga and Chinese Taoism.

When there is sufficient inner silence present via the daily practice of deep meditation, and then the breath and body are brought into the process via spinal breathing pranayama, asanas, mudras, bandhas, and tantric sexual methods, we will notice three things occurring.

1. An expansion of sexual energy from the pelvic region upward, with part finding its way into the GI tract.

2. The natural retention of air in the GI tract.

3. The interaction of food with the sexual essences and air in the GI tract.

The natural combination of these three elements in the digestive system through an emerging higher form of digestion gives rise to a new substance emanating from the GI tract, which permeates the entire body. Much of this penetration occurs as this substance enters the spinal canal and rises up through the chest cavity to the head. The highly penetrating and sometimes intoxicating substance produced in the GI tract has been given many names. A name prevalent in yoga is *soma*. The word *soma* also refers to a hallucinogenic plant, which is not what we are talking about here. In Taoism, the GI tract, when engaged in this higher functioning, is called the *caldron*, recognizing the alchemy that is occurring there – three ordinary substances (sexual essence, air, and food) being combined to create an extraordinary substance that is a key to the process of human spiritual transformation.

The process continues in the head, with further refinements occurring in the brain, which lead to another substance being secreted through the sinuses, down through the inside nasal passages, into the throat and then down into the GI tract again, where it joins in the process already described. This recycling of subtle essences leads to even more refined processing in the GI tract. The substance coming down from the brain into the GI tract is referred to as *amrita* (nectar) in the yoga tradition. It can sometimes be experienced as a sweet aroma in the nasal passages and taste in the mouth.

The overall experience of this combining and transformation of substances, and the recycling of the resulting essences in the body leads to large flows of ecstatic pleasure throughout the body, and the radiation of energy beyond the body. This is why those who are advancing in spiritual practices are sometimes said to be *radiant*. There is a specific neurobiology behind it. In yogic terms, the body-wide radiance of ecstatic energy indicates the rise of the mythical quality of *ojas*, which is a greatly enhanced manifestation of vitality that is easily noticed by others.

If we begin to understand that such a process really exists and, better yet, begin to experience aspects of it within ourselves as a result of our daily practices, then we are able to look at diet from an entirely new angle. And we can also see the relevance of shatkarmas (cleansing techniques) and amaroli (urine therapy) as well. All of these methods are aimed at enhancing and optimizing the process just described.

As mentioned earlier, diet is not a core practice in yoga, but an important supporting element. If we look at this that way, we can see how our cooperation with inner urges relating to diet can enhance the overall process that is occurring on the road to enlightenment.

The higher form of digestion described above can generate a lot of heat in the GI tract, radiating out to fill the whole body. It is sometimes referred to as the *kundalini fire*. When the fires are burning, it can be beneficial to eat heavier foods more often. Then the fire (intense digestive activity) can be used to consume the substances in our GI tract in a more regulated way to produce more *soma*, rather than frying us from the inside, which is the sensation we can get sometimes if eating too lightly when energy is surging within us. It is also possible to quench the inner fires and related inner energy imbalances with application of the diet methods of *Ayurveda*, which take into account our bodily constitution and inner energy flows, and how certain foods can either aggravate or pacify these. See the appendix for more on ayurvedic diet guidelines.

To keep it as simple as possible, we just listen to what we are being called to do from within with respect to our diet, and in other aspects of our daily activity. When we are engaged in daily deep meditation, we may feel inclined to eat a lighter diet. And when our kundalini becomes active, we may feel inclined to eat a heavier diet at times, and a lighter diet at other times. It will depend on the energy dynamics occurring within us, and the process of purification and opening that is underway.

We learn to become good listeners to the inner voice of our neurobiology as we travel the road to enlightenment.

Food Preparation and Consumption

While there are numerous approaches to diet, there are only so many ways to cook our food. We can bake it, broil it, boil it, barbecue it, fry it, steam it, marinate it, or eat it raw.

Of course, there are thousands of variations on these few methods, in terms of what to cook when, how, and with what. Still, it will be the basic ingredients that make the difference in the end. The ingredients we put into our cooking are, more or less, what will end up on the plate, and in us.

There is also another factor. The way we cook our food can change the character of the ingredients we are using, and their nutritional content. For example, if we are barbecuing shish kabob with fresh fruits and vegetables on a stick, and mistakenly burn the whole thing until it is black, is it going to be the same food we started with? Obviously not. It will not even be edible. Likewise, if we boil our food until much of its nutritional content is dissolved in the water, this will not be ideal either, unless we plan on consuming the water along with the food. Even then, it may be too late to gain any nutritional benefit from the enzymes we have destroyed in the cooking process. There are ways we can cook our food too much, losing some or all of the nutritional benefit of what we started with. So, is the answer to eat all of our food raw? Some believe this, adhering to a strict raw food diet. In this case, the choice may be usually for fruits, vegetables and nuts only. With such diets, slicing, grinding and juicing may be the only ways to achieve good variety and nutrition.

But there is a middle ground, you know, somewhere between cooking our food too much and not cooking it at all. It is in the middle where it is suggested to look. In that broad range of options, we can find many ways to prepare our food, while preserving good nutrition through a wide variety of foods.

So, if we are going to barbecue, let us remember not to over do it (obviously), or underdo it either. If we are boiling our food, let's keep in mind that boiling pulls the nutrients out of vegetables, especially long boiling with a lot of water. So maybe better to boil our rice and pasta and go another route with our vegetables.

Frying and broiling with very little fat are good in moderation, as is baking for foods that are conducive to these methods.

Steaming is an excellent way to cook most vegetables, since it does not add fat and achieves the cooking while preserving the nutritional value much better than boiling. Of course, a raw food advocate would not find steaming acceptable either. So we each have to go with our own preferences. The more rigid we are in our selection of food and preparation style, the more limited our options will be, and this can actually end up costing us by leading us toward a less balanced diet. Limiting selection will eventually catch up with us. This is why fad diets of any kind are not recommended.

The herd will seldom be right when it comes to diet and food preparation. This is because healthy eating is not determined primarily through intellect. It is determined by listening to the needs of our body at its present level of functioning and in relation to the foods that are available to it. Our intellect can serve this listening, but it cannot lead it effectively. Diet is not ruled by ideology. It is ruled by biology. And our biology is constantly changing, especially if we are on a path involving effective spiritual practices.

So, our diet preferences are going to be changing over time, and so will our cooking and food consumption preferences. That is why it is good to be familiar with the middle ground, and to favor moderation in all things. Then, as our preferences change, we will be less likely to be running off on unhealthy tangents. This is true with many things in life, isn't it? It is certainly true with yoga practices. And it is true in matters of diet as well.

The lot of variety can also be found in the preferences people have on how often to eat. While those with a hypoglycemic (unstable blood sugar) tendency may feel encouraged to eat small meals often throughout the day, others might eat only one larger meal each day. In the middle is the "breakfast, lunch and dinner" crowd, which represents the majority of people. There is no right or wrong in this. Each of us will find the right frequency of eating that suits our unique nature, and where we happen to be on our spiritual path.

As we prepare and consume our food each day, it is good to remember that food plays an important role, not only in our basic nutrition, but also in the spiritual processes that are unfolding within us. As our spiritual neurobiology awakens, our dietary requirements may change, as well as how we prepare our food and how often we eat.

As we engage in food preparation and food consumption, let's remember the inner divine role we are fostering within ourselves. Whatever our spiritual or religious beliefs may be, we can be thankful for the grace that is bestowed on us, and offer the food we prepare and eat for the expansion of happiness in all we do and for everyone on the earth.

Eating Habits, Addictions and Flights of Fancy

All that we accomplish in life is based on the formation of habits. We are creatures of habit, and this can be used to great advantage. On the other side of the coin, we can fall into habits that are not in our best interest. So much of what we do to improve our lot in life is directly related to how we manage our habits.

If we have begun a spiritual practice like deep meditation, our success with the practice will not depend on how pleasant an experience we might have today, tomorrow or the next day. It will depend on our ability to sustain our daily practice over months and years, through all the ups and downs we will be sure to experience along the way. It will be our habit that will carry us through.

Inner Silence and Eating Habits

The same is true with our diet. The eating habits we form and live with will influence our health and our progress in spiritual practices.

If we are engaged in deep meditation, we will have inner silence coming from within, and this will aid us greatly in making adjustments in our habits in what we eat, and when and how we eat it. We may find ourselves eating lighter more nutritious foods, taking our time doing it, and chewing our food much better. In fact, it can be said that the rise of inner silence is a primary influence in lifting all of our habits up to support increasing levels of health and happiness in all avenues of life.

As we are growing inside, we will find ourselves much more able to act on information and methods we encounter on the outside. What is true will ring true more readily as we grow from within, and we will find the strength to reprogram our ingrained habits to operate on a higher level. This is the primary dynamic involved in improving our life in all areas.

With inner silence comes a greater faith in our ability to change, to grow, and to expand in joy and love. As we become more aware, we can overcome our old habits and cultivate new ones that enable us to forge ahead in life. It has been said that those who have the desire to change can. The rise of inner silence elevates our desires and our ability to act on them in the direction of permanent positive change.

Of course, raw willpower can be used to accomplish things also. But willpower alone will eventually tire if it is not rooted in our steady stillness, and in our connection within ourselves to something greater than the limits of times and space. The source of steadfast willpower is inner silence.

Habit is what determines our actions in life, and rising inner silence is what gives us the ability to lift our habits to a higher plane.

Addictions

What is addiction? In the simplest definition, addiction is a habit we are unable or unwilling to change. There are addictions that can be beneficial, such as an addiction to divine unfoldment, without limiting its scope in any way. It can also be seen as an unwavering dedication to a cause – an obsession. Some might not see this as good. Yet, an addiction to divine unfoldment will eventually lead to its own transcendence. It is an addiction to surrender, an addiction to letting go – one of the essential secrets of devotion in spiritual matters. It is *active surrender*.

On the other hand there are addictions that will retard our spiritual progress and can hold us back from progress in many areas of life. These are addictions that sustain and add to the obstructions to inner silence within us. These may be considered to be chemical or psychological. The most destructive addictions are a combination of both. A destructive addiction is one that gives us a false sense of wellbeing, while holding us back from real progress at the same time.

In terms of the things we eat, such addictions can take many forms:

- Alcohol

- Tobacco

- Caffeine

- Refined Sugar

- Medicine and food supplements

- Chronic overeating of any or all foods

- Chronic undereating of all foods (anorexia)

Any of the items mentioned, approached in moderation, will not be harmful. In fact, the road to health and happiness is paved with moderation in all things.

On the other hand, any food or substance that is consumed compulsively to excess (even water) can be regarded as a negative addiction. On the other side of it, an obsession with consuming less can be a negative addiction also (anorexia). Many addictions are not recognized and are perpetuating themselves through subconsciously ingrained obsessive habits. We all have them. Much of our spiritual progress is related to the unwinding of obsessive conduct, which retards our natural growth.

How do we overcome negative additions? The same way we overcome any habits, eating or other, that hold us back from health and happiness. It is always going to be an inner journey leading to surrender to that which is evolutionary and positive within us. Yoga practices are designed for this. They clean the mud off the windshield of our nervous system, so all will become gradually much more clear, and we can navigate through life with more clarity and purpose.

In the case of strong negative addictions, yoga practices may not be enough. In that case, we have the option to resort to more direct means to overcome compulsive negative habits. The twelve-step program, originally developed by Alcoholics Anonymous, is the most effective known means for dealing with a strong negative addiction. It has been expanded to cover every kind of compulsive and addictive behavior. The twelve-step program is a kind of yoga. It involves admitting that we cannot change by ourselves, and surrendering to a *higher power*. As soon as we are able to do this in any avenue of our life, great power surges up to aid us in our time of trouble. The twelve-step program is a specialized way of applying the principles of desire and surrender to overcome negative addiction, leading to a happier healthier life.

Flights of Fancy

There is the idea out there that if a little of something is good for us, then a lot of it will be even better. Some take it to the point that if we do nothing but that one thing, then this will surely deliver us from all that ails us, and bring us (and the entire world!) enlightenment as well. Unfortunately, it doesn't work that way. This sort of obsessive conduct can be called the *magic bullet syndrome*, or a *flight of fancy*.

To make steady progress in life, it takes a broad-based application of spiritual practices supporting a gradual move toward all around healthful living habits. The *magic bullet* approach to designing a better diet and lifestyle is a manifestation of the same compulsive behavior we find behind negative addictions. It is compounded by the rational mind assuming that the more of this thing we do the better off we will be. In a sense, the tendency to pursue flights of fancy is more problematic than a recognized negative addiction. A flight of fancy can go on for a long time. When it finally does crash, many reasons for its failure can be conjured up and assigned elsewhere, and the person involved in it may then move on to the next magic bullet flight of fancy. It is similar to a negative addiction. Some of us go through all of life like this, seeking the holy grail, not knowing that the holy grail is in us all along, found in a steady moderate approach encompassing an integration of effective spiritual methods and the sound lifestyle choices that will be the natural result.

Getting some sunshine on a regular basis can be healthful. Is lying in the sun (or staring at the sun) for hours at a time healthful? No it isn't.

Taking a few vitamin supplements each day can enhance our nutrition. Will taking ten, or twenty, or fifty vitamin supplements each day enhance our nutrition? Maybe, and quite possibly bring a host of undesirable side effects as well, including some that may seriously compromise our health.

Likewise, the judicious use of prescription and non-prescription drugs can alleviate suffering and extend life. But do we need a drug for every hiccup we may experience? The aggressive marketing programs of the drug companies tell us we do (for their own reasons), but we know better in our inner silence.

Obviously, it is good to consult professionals when considering utilizing supplements and drug prescriptions, especially if we suspect a serious health issue. However, if it reaches the point where we are shoveling pills in our mouth to compensate for an unhealthy lifestyle, or we are taking drugs to treat side effects from other drugs, then something is seriously wrong. It is the *flight of fancy* out of control. It can happen in the most professional environments. Flights of fancy are not limited to individuals. They can run rampant in our institutions as well.

We can see that even in the most health-oriented endeavors, excess can creep in, leading to diminishing returns. This can be as great an obstacle to our health and spiritual progress as any other kind of unhealthful living.

Halluncinogenics and Yoga

In the native cultures of the world (including in ancient India), spiritual experience has sometimes been associated (and ritualized) with the ingestion of hallucinogenic substances derived from plants. In modern times, the use of such substances for recreational purposes has become common, especially marijuana, certain types of mushrooms, and synthetic substances, particularly LSD, which rose to prominence in the youth *counter culture* of the 1960s and 1970s. Many from that era give some credit to their drug experiences in helping launch them on serious and drugless spiritual paths later on. It cannot be denied. This leaves us with two lingering questions.

First, are drug experiences necessary to embark on a spiritual path? The answer is obviously, no, for many pursue spiritual awakening without a drug experience being the initial stimulus. However, it can be said that in many cases, some sort of initial altered state of consciousness led to the inspiration and desire for a more permanent awakening. Such an initial experience can be caused by an accident, an illness, a spontaneous inner awakening, spiritual vision, or other life-altering event. Or maybe the aspirant just knows inside that there is something more to life than the conventional knowledge society is offering. The seed of spiritual desire can germinate from many causes. Ultimately, the call comes from within.

Drugs are only one of many ways people can be inspired to pursue a broader possibility within. In virtually all cases where an initial altered state is experienced, it will only be a preview, and not the onset of permanent spiritual transformation. It is important to recognize that any particular spiritual experience does not constitute a final outcome. For moving toward a final outcome in terms of spiritual progress, a different strategy is necessary, one which will systematically and gradually promote the purification and opening of the nervous system to its full capabilities.

This leads to the second question: Are drugs an aid in ongoing yoga practice? If there is any initial benefit found in the artificial experience produced by drugs, then the repetition of that experience is not likely to take us further. To assume so is yet another flight of fancy – the magic bullet syndrome. In the case of continuing with hallucinogenic drugs to recreate a particular kind of experience, we will be producing the opposite effect underneath – adding to the obstructions lodged deep within our nervous system.

Spiritual development is not primarily about having a temporary peak experience. Rather, it is a natural and permanent awakening, which can be achieved only through ongoing deep inner purification. This is why anyone engaged in daily deep meditation will find urges for substances that produce artificial experiences falling away. This applies to hallucinogenic drugs, alcohol, tobacco, caffeine, and eating habits that retard the natural expression of the divine light emerging from within us.

Fasting

Restricting or eliminating food intake for a time, known as *fasting*, is an ancient practice that can be found in most of the world's spiritual traditions. These days, it has been ritualized in the religions to the point of being little more than an occasional ceremonial observance. Yet, there is great value hidden in fasting that is being rediscovered in modern times as more people have sought to reveal the underlying truths in their religion and the effectiveness of spiritual methods that have been utilized by serious practitioners for thousands of years.

The principle behind fasting is simple. When the body is given an opportunity to take a break from processing food, it will purify itself. Its energy resources are naturally redirected from digestion and assimilation, and are fully devoted to conducting an inner cleanup. In this mode, the body is much better able to overcome disease and obstructions in the organs, tissues and nervous system, including the subtle neurobiological blockages within us that are the primary inhibitors of our spiritual unfoldment. So, prudent fasting is both an effective health therapy and an important spiritual practice, all rolled into one.

Fasting is an aspect of *diet*, because diet is not only about what we are eating, but also about what we are not eating. While, in the strictest sense, fasting is about not eating anything for a period of time, the *fasting effect*, can also be observed to be working to one degree or another across the entire range of our dietary habits. In other words, the health and spiritual benefits of eating a light and nutritious diet are due in large part to the *fasting effect*, which is a condition of inner functioning that provides the natural processes of the body a greater opportunity to engage in cleansing, purification and opening.

So, while a purist may regard anything more than zero food consumption to not be fasting, we are more interested in the practical results that can be achieved by moderating food intake to varying degrees at different times. This brings us back into our main diet discussion, which is about what we are doing with food every day, whether we are doing a full blown fast, or simply favoring lighter more nutritious eating habits. Both will be stimulating the fasting effect to varying degrees.

The goal in the AYP system is to effectively utilize all of the known principles of human spiritual transformation through the integration and optimization of effective practices. This will, by necessity, draw us away from extremist attitudes about any particular spiritual method. As with diet, attitudes about fasting that we see in the world may also have a tendency toward an extreme *magic bullet* mentality and *flights of fancy*, with the corresponding loss of focus on maintaining a balanced approach. The extreme approaches we may encounter as we explore these methods do not invalidate the usefulness of the underlying principles themselves. We just need to find a rational moderate approach.

Those who pursue extreme approaches can distort the real value to be found in the method they may be fanatically promoting. Let's not be swayed by extreme points of view, and take the middle road that takes good advantage of sound principles of spiritual transformation leading to steady progress with safety.

We began with sound spiritual practices like deep meditation and spinal breathing pranayama. And then we discussed the natural emergence of healthful and spiritually evolutionary eating habits. We make choices about these things as our awareness expands from within and as our neurobiology naturally seeks a higher mode of functioning. It is the same when we consider fasting. We have been moving in that direction already.

There are several ways to approach fasting. It will depend on our personal preferences, and also on our metabolic health when starting out.

The simplest way to add more of the *fasting effect* into our daily routine is to skip a meal for several days running. Our ability to do so will depend largely on our comfort level. For some, it will be very uncomfortable and difficult. For others, fairly easy. It is a good place to start with our own experiment in fasting. Skipping a meal does not mean eating twice as much at the next meal. It means reducing the total food intake for a day, one meal's worth, or for several days if we find it to be comfortable.

For those with a medical condition such as hypoglycemia or diabetes, where reducing food consumption could be hazardous, a doctor should be consulted before undertaking any sort of fast.

The advantage of the meal skipping approach is that it is easy for almost anyone to do anytime, to begin experiencing the fasting effect. The disadvantage in the meal skipping approach is that we may notice discomfort expressing itself as *hunger*. With a fast involving no food for several days or more, the discomfort is generally found not to be hunger, because it passes. Then we know it for what it is – the biological withdrawal symptoms associated with a habitual dependence on food intake. No one will starve in a few days or even a few weeks without food. But many have felt like they were starving, due to the withdrawal symptoms associated with no food intake after only a few hours. Interestingly, those who are on a long fast don't feel hungry, once the initial adjustment has occurred. For those who have experience with fasting for several days or more, the discomfort passes until much later when a genuine hunger returns. This latter stage hunger is a signal that a fast may be ended naturally.

Liquids are another matter. No fast should ever be undertaken without adequate hydration. Our body needs water on a daily basis to continue to function, whether we are fasting or not. On a strict fast, only water is necessary to continue it. There is also the popular juice fast, which adds nutrients, particularly sugar, which is an energy source. For those who are inclined toward ongoing discomfort during a fast, a juice fast may be preferable.

We each will find our own balance. For many of us, moving gradually to a light and nutritious diet may be more than enough. This too involves the fasting effect – lightening the food processing load in the body so our energies can better support our inner processes of purification and opening, and also the production of refined substances directly related to our emerging enlightenment.

This brings up the matter of kundalini again, which is the rise of ecstatic conductivity and radiance in our body, facilitated by the associated refinements in digestion.

If we are adjusting to an awakening kundalini, we should follow the diet guidelines mentioned earlier, which will at times lean toward a heavier diet and eating more often to temper the fire in the GI tract. During this stage of our inner development, fasting will not be advisable, as it can accelerate the purification process and exacerbate our kundalini symptoms.

Fasting is most useful before we have awakened our inner energies, and then later on when our higher neurobiology has stabilized. During the in-between period of kundalini energy awakening and adjustment, we will be wise to adjust our eating habits to support that. There is a time for everything, and everything in its own time.

In cases of illness, fasting can be combined with Amaroli (urine therapy) to apply the powerful combined natural healing effects provided by these two practices. This is discussed in Chapter 4.

Fasting may also be combined with sun gazing and breathing techniques, which profess to provide the means for sustaining life from sunlight and air, without food intake. Whether this is true or not remains to be investigated by modern science. If such abilities exist within us, we may find signs of their manifestation as a result of long term yoga practice. Focusing on such phenomena to the exclusion of deep meditation, spinal breathing pranayama and other yoga practices will likely be premature. Let's be mindful of our tendency to get caught up in *flights of fancy*.

The blessing of self-directed and self-paced spiritual practice is that we can make adjustments in our practices as necessary to accommodate our inner unfoldment. This applies to the evolution of our diet over the long term, and to the judicious use of fasting according to our preferences and needs.

The Body-Mind-Spirit Connection

We know from modern physics that there is nothing here except miniscule bits of energy polarity interacting with each other to form the appearance and substance of this world we are familiar with. Likewise the scriptures of the world, in one terminology or another, point to omnipresent unmanifest spirit permeating and upholding all that is manifest.

There is really nothing here at all. And yet, here we are going about the daily business of our lives. It is a mystery.

While many have borne witness over the centuries to the profound benefits of realizing our spiritual nature, many of us remain somewhat unconvinced, even as our vast religious institutions stand as constant reminders (albeit, distorted at times) of what sages and prophets have lived and shared over the centuries.

The message is simple. We are eternal spirit, manifesting through body and mind. In our hearts we know this is true, for it is in the heart where we are joined in *Oneness*, and directly experience that we are constantly connected in body, mind and spirit.

Within the human body, there are numerous processes at work that will naturally support our evolution toward full realization, if we but encourage them to do so. This is the essence of yoga, the application of a range of methods leading to full expression of spirit through us. It has been called the emergence of *stillness in action*, or the rise *of outpouring of divine love*. This is our destiny as we travel the evolutionary scale.

The food we eat has a direct relationship to our evolution. While it is not the primary means for spiritual transformation, food plays an important supporting role, especially as we become more advanced on our path. We cannot force our evolution by changing our diet, but we can enhance our progress by heeding the inner call.

As we rise in our sensitivity through daily deep meditation, we will hear the call and adjust our habits in ways that can dramatically enhance our realization of the mind/body/spirit connection. In time, we will come to know that this connection encompasses everyone and everything. Through direct experience, we come to know ourselves as that *Oneness*, and we conduct ourselves accordingly in our daily affairs, serving the greater good as we serve our own.

Chapter 3 – Shatkarmas for Cleansing

The primary yoga practices we may choose to undertake include deep meditation, spinal breathing pranayama, asanas, mudras, bandhas and others. These (meditation especially) will elicit a call from within us, which can lead us to a purer, healthier diet. In addition, we may also feel called to engage in physical methods which will further purify our body and nervous system. Indeed, asanas, mudras, bandhas, and even pranayama (breathing techniques) fall into this category, and may be stimulated into action by deep meditation alone.

The shatkarmas are specific cleansing techniques that are targeted toward the inner channels of the body, particularly the gastrointestinal (GI) tract, nasal passages and sinuses, which have a significant impact on the flow of neurobiological (ecstatic) energy throughout the body. Shatkarmas also include our normal hygiene related to bathing and cleaning of the eyes, ears and mouth. These will not be discussed very much here, as it is assumed everyone has a basic hygienic routine already. What will be covered in detail are methods that may not be so familiar, which go significantly beyond basic hygiene as exercised in modern culture.

There is some overlap between the shatkarmas and other aspects of yoga such as mudras, bandhas and pranayama. The main difference will be in the ability we have to incorporate a practice into our asanas and sitting practices routine, versus flushing the inner passages of the body with water, which will usually take place in the bathroom. It is these shatkarmas we will focus on mainly, since they provide significant enhancements for our purification and opening, in addition to the many practices we have already covered in the AYP writings.

The shatkarmas we will cover here include:

- Jala Neti (nasal wash)

- Basti (colon cleansing/enema)

- Dhauti (intestinal wash)

Additional shatkarmas will be discussed in relation to our daily routine of yoga practices. These include Nauli (churning of the abdominal muscles), Kapalbhati (sudden exhale, a nerve cleansing pranayama method), and Trataka (an eye/attention gazing method).

All of the shatkarmas have a profound relationship to our overall routine of yoga practices. Before we get into the techniques themselves, let's see how shatkarmas relate in general to our full program of practices, and to our emerging enlightenment.

Bodily Purification and Enlightenment

It has been said that the human body is the *City of God*. We can also say that the human body, and the nervous system in particular, is a *window to the divine*. Yoga practices are designed to aid in cleaning the window so the full light of our inner divine qualities can shine through. This is experienced as increasing inner peace, creativity, energy, and a more illuminated view of the world. That is why the end stage of the purification and opening process is called *enlightenment*.

Can this purification and opening be accomplished through physical means alone? No. Physical measures such as the diet and cleansing methods described in this book, and in other AYP books on postures (asanas), mudras, bandhas, tantric sexual practices, etc., cover the physical (energetic) side of our purification and opening. It runs much deeper than that, and that is why spiritual desire (bhakti), deep meditation, spinal breathing pranayama, and other methods involving heart, mind and breath receive much attention in the overall scheme of our yoga practices. The non-physical methods of yoga reach far deeper than the physical methods.

On the other hand, physical methods are an essential part of the broad scope of yoga as summarized in Patanjali's *eight limbs of yoga*.

There is always the question of what to do first as we build our yoga practice routine. In the AYP approach we begin with deep meditation and spinal breathing pranayama before we move into more physical methods. With this orientation, the urge to engage in physical methods may emerge automatically. It is not uncommon for those who are engaged in daily deep meditation to naturally favor a lighter more nutritious diet, better hygiene, and even yoga postures and inner physical maneuvers (mudras and bandhas). We call this *automatic yoga*, which is inspired by the rise of inner silence. It is evidence that all of the limbs of yoga are resident within us and naturally connected. Activate one limb of yoga, and all the others will be stimulated. The deeper the method we choose to engage in (such as deep meditation) the more the other limbs will be stimulated.

Depending on where we are on our path of purification and opening, physical methods such as the shatkarmas, can play a greater or lesser role in our opening. For example, if we are on the verge of an energy awakening, or entering into one, shatkarmas can become very important. This is because our inner physical channels are then transforming to a higher level of functioning, and cleansing in the nasal passages, sinuses and GI tract will enhance these refined processes. So we may feel a strong urge to engage in shatkarmas at that time.

Shatkarmas may also be undertaken for health reasons. There is no doubt that a full range of yoga practices, including shatkarmas, can be a great benefit to our physical health.

Taking proactive measures with diet and shatkarmas can jump start inner progress in the early stages of our deep meditation practice. After a few months of daily deep meditation, if not much seems to be happening in the way of positive effects in our daily activity, then diet and shatkarma measures may help. Of course, this can only result if there is a strong spiritual desire (bhakti) emerging from within to engage in these additional measures, which is a sign that deep meditation is working to elevate our longing for progress.

<u>All yoga practices are connected within us.</u>

So, whether we are inclined toward doing shatkarmas now or later, we can be sure it will be in concert with our spiritual desires, deep meditation and other practices we are engaged in. And, likewise, as we undertake shatkarmas, this too will have a stimulating effect on our other practices.

In many cases, shatkarmas may not be undertaken at all. There is no rule that says all practitioners of yoga must engage in all aspects of yoga. We will know when we are being called, by the symptoms and urges that come from within us. Some practices we may never be inclined to undertake, and that is okay. If we are finding good progress and more happiness and fulfillment in our life, that is all that matters.

The urge to engage in shatkarmas may be strong at one time on our path, and then wane later on, as our nervous system becomes more self-sufficient in sustaining the higher functioning associated with ecstatic conductivity and radiance (kundalini). In this sense, shatkarmas are different from deep meditation, spinal breathing pranayama and some of our other practices, which we may continue with on a daily basis for a lifetime. Shatkarmas may be needed in the beginning or the middle, but not often near the end of our journey. Shatkarmas can be viewed to be a kind of *training wheel* for our inner ecstatic processes. As these processes come into their own, we may be less inclined to use the training wheel. This can happen with diet also, which is less critical in the end than it may be in the beginning or middle stages of our spiritual journey.

Great sages have occasionally de-emphasized the rigorous diet obsessions of those with less experience and development, going so far as to demonstrate that they could eat almost anything without ill effects.

One size does not fit all in matters of diet and shatkarmas, and it is largely a matter of hearing our own inner calling along the way on the path and utilizing these methods as inwardly inspired. Our inclinations will likely change as our purification and opening advances over time, first to more attention on diet and shatkarmas, and perhaps eventually to less attention on these things as we move on to the glories of abiding inner silence, ecstatic bliss, and outpouring divine love.

Then, the call we hear most of the time will be for radiating joy everywhere in the form of service to others, and the constant inquiry into our infinite unifying nature. All of our yoga practices are stepping-stones to that. All are methods of purification leading to enlightenment.

Cleansing of Mouth, Nasal Passages and Sinuses

Whether we are looking to improve our health, or advance our spiritual progress, cleansing of the mouth, nasal passages and sinuses can be an important activity. Not everyone will need to do this beyond the basic methods of oral hygiene, but it is good to know that we can do more as the need arises.

Once the nervous system is ready to begin to open ecstatically (kundalini), cleansing in the nasal passages and sinuses can become especially significant. The neurobiology of the brain as influenced by mudras such as sambhavi and kechari tie in with this also. So there is a higher purpose to these cleansing methods.

Mouth and Tongue

We have all been brought up (hopefully) to practice good oral hygiene by brushing our teeth every day and flossing regularly to remove tartar (plaque) from our teeth. There are varying opinions on using antiseptic mouthwashes, so it is suggested to go with the intuition on that. Our habits of oral hygiene will improve as we advance in yoga.

A yoga method that can be added to daily oral hygiene, which few may be exposed to in modern society, is *tongue scraping*. Sometimes brushing the tongue with the toothbrush is advised after brushing the teeth. The yogic equivalent of this is tongue scraping, which is far more effective for removing tartar and its resident bacteria from the tongue. This involves using the edge of a straight piece of metal or plastic to scrape the top of the tongue forward from the area right in front of the taste buds. A more effective tool for this is a flat strip of metal that has been bent into a "U" shape. The curved edge can be used to scrape forward on the top of the tongue, covering the full top surface with a single stroke, or several repetitions.

The amount of tartar collected with tongue scraping in this manner will far exceed what can be accomplished with a brush, and will greatly reduce the amount of tartar collecting on the teeth as well.

Of course, excessive tartar on the tongue and teeth can be a sign of an imbalance in the diet and/or general health condition. If that is the case, we can step back further and look at our lifestyle to address the root causes of excess proteins and bacteria (tartar) building up in the mouth. If we do this, we will find ourselves with a much cleaner mouth, and much better all around health as well.

The condition of our mouth at any point in time is a visible indication of the condition of the rest of our body, and the quality of life we have been living.

Nasal Passages and Sinuses – Neti Pot

The nasal passages and sinuses play a key role in the neurobiology of human spiritual transformation and the rise to enlightenment. It is through this region that an intimate connection between the brain and the rest of the nervous system occurs. So daily cleansing of the nasal passages and sinuses may be desirable at certain times along our path. We will know intuitively when it is time for this. There are also significant health benefits to be found in knowing how to cleanse these delicate tissues.

The age-old yogic method for cleansing the nasal passages and sinuses is called *jala neti*, or *nasal wash*, which is running salted water through in a safe and comfortable way. Several mudras and pranayama methods work in the nasal passages and sinuses also, without using water. These include *yoni mudra*, *kechari mudra*, *sambhavi mudra*, *bastrika pranayama*, and *kapalbhati* (below).

The simplest way to begin to do jala neti is with a *neti pot*, which is like a small teapot with a spout that fits comfortably into the nostril. It is easily obtained through any yoga supply store. With appropriately mixed salty water in the neti pot and the spout inserted in one nostril with face turned down over the sink, then the head is turned to the side so the water will run into the nostril. From there it will run through the nasal passage, over the back edge of the nasal septum (the divider between left and right nostrils), and back out through the other nostril and into the sink, as illustrated here:

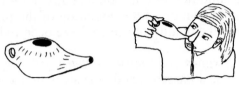

Use of a Neti Pot

This is first done through one nostril, and then through the other nostril. The order does not matter. As long as the head is tipped forward during this procedure, no water will find its way into the throat. A little might spill over into the mouth, and that can be easily expelled through the mouth. (See the next section on doing jala neti using a bowl.)

In the course of doing this easy procedure with a neti pot, the sinuses will also be filled with the saline solution, gently massaging and cleansing them. Once both nostrils have received and emptied the neti pot, and have drained, it will take a few minutes more to drain the sinuses. This is done by slowly tilting the head to the left and the right, and then up and down over the sink. Water will continue to come out of the sinuses for a few minutes, so be patient. If you walk out of the bathroom too soon, you may end up draining your sinuses on the living room rug!

The amount of salt we put in the water is important, as this determines the comfort (or lack of it) we will find in doing jala neti.

Obviously, if the practice gives us discomfort, we will not be inclined to do it. So getting the salt content right is essential. Everyone will be a little different in this, so some trial and error will probably be necessary to get the salt content just right for you.

Slightly warm tap water can be used, if the water is sanitary. It is preferred to use pure salt without additives, such as iodine. One to two teaspoons per quart or liter of water is a range of concentration, which translates to about one-half to one teaspoon per pint or half liter. For a small neti pot, few pinches of salt will be adequate.

Adjustments to salt content are made based on how it feels going through our nostrils. Everyone is a little different in this, and the above ranges are approximate. If there is too much or too little salt, there can be stinging sensations or other signs of discomfort, and we should adjust our salt content accordingly. No permanent damage will result from using incorrect salt concentration, but it isn't fun either, so we should make the necessary adjustments. When the salt content is right for us, there will *be no discomfort at all* as the water passes through our sensitive nasal and sinus tissues. This is how we will know we have the correct salt content. Experiment and see for yourself.

It is like that with many yoga practices. The most comfortable application of a yoga practice is usually the best application. Always self-pace for that.

Jala neti can be performed daily as part of our morning hygiene, or as needed. For more advanced practitioners, the neti pot may be replaced with a bowl. Jala neti may also be combined with amaroli (discussed in the next chapter).

Nasal Passages and Sinuses – Water Bowl

Once we have mastered the neti pot, we may feel like we'd like to have a more thorough cleansing of our nasal passages and sinuses. This will mean using more water than can be delivered at one time with the small neti pot. Of course, we can keep refilling the neti pot and run as much water through as we like. There is also another way, which is using a bowl instead of neti pot, and drawing the water up directly through our nasal passages with negative pressure from the lungs, rather than a neti pot, which relies on gravity to pass water through the nasal passages.

Using a bowl for jala neti is a more advanced procedure, but not nearly as difficult or risky as it might seem when first considering it.

It can be a pretty short trip from the neti pot to sucking salted warm water up from a bowl with both nostrils and expelling it through the mouth. The bowl can be emptied in a few cycles this way. The water can also be expelled through the nose, but that is messier. The nasal pharynx is a natural vessel for this operation, and even has a "dam" in the form of the soft palate inhibiting the water from running down into the throat while inhaling it up through the nose, which is the same effect as when using the neti pot.

Using the bowl is fast and effective. The longest part of it is waiting for the sinuses to drain, which can take a few minutes. That is true of any form of jala neti, but especially when doing a whole bowl, which can be a pint (half-liter) or more of water.

If this form of jala neti sounds risky, it isn't. With this procedure, the instances of inhaling water will be practically non-existent. We have a natural ability to handle water in this way. But if the salt content is too much or too little, it will not be so pleasant, so do mind the instructions above for getting the salt content adjusted just right for comfort.

Colon Cleansing

It has been said that many diseases can be cured through colon cleansing – the use of enemas. Hence the rise in popularity of this practice, and even the springing up of *colon cleansing clinics* across the landscape. Like with so many things in yoga, a moderate approach can be very helpful for our spiritual progress and health. But an obsession with any one practice at the expense of everything else can be counter-productive. It is with that warning that we discuss colon cleansing, or *basti*.

The colon is the part of the intestines that goes from the appendix in the lower right abdomen upward (ascending), across from right to left just above the navel (transverse), and back down (descending) the left side of the abdomen to the rectum and the anus.

Basti is a simple warm water enema with a gravity bag, hose with clamp, and an insert fitting at the end, which fits in the anus.

Enema Bag

Slightly warm tap water can be used if it is free of bacteria. If not, use bottled water. No salt is used. With the bag hung a few feet above the anus, carefully fill up the colon with about a quart or liter of water (or less), either leaning forward on the toilet or lying down on the left side. To protect against urinary tract infection, care should be taken not to leak water from the anus on to the urethra – ladies especially. Wait for a few minutes before expelling. Some light nauli (described later in this chapter) can be done while sitting on the toilet before and during the emptying of the colon. This easy and quick procedure will provide a good colon clean-out.

For spiritual purposes basti can be done every morning before bathing and sitting practices, along with jala neti/nasal wash. However, this is not a routine for beginning yoga practitioners, nor needed for advanced practitioners with ecstatic conductivity well established. The shatkarmas are most useful for spiritual purposes in the middle stage cultivation of ecstatic conductivity, done in conjunction with a full yoga routine.

For health reasons, one might prefer to use basti for relief during times of stress, constipation and other digestive problems.

Can basti become a habit that we cannot let go of, so we become dependent on the enema to clear our bowels? Not necessarily. Basti can be used daily for spiritual purposes for a long time in support of the yoga routine to assist the awakening of ecstatic conductivity. Then, at some point when ecstatic awakening has become strong and self-sustaining, basti can be discontinued and used only occasionally thereafter.

With the many changes in neurobiological functioning that occur in advancing yoga, regular elimination becomes part of the overall ecstatic neurobiology, but it takes a transition (with a full range of practices) to get there. The cleansing shatkarmas, including basti, are part of that transitional phase.

So there is no rush to begin basti and shatkarmas in general if we are new to yoga. It is much better to become established in deep meditation, spinal breathing pranayama and other yoga practices, and then the shatkarmas will be there when we need them. We will know when to take them up, based on our inner leanings, just as we will know when and how our diet may change as inner development advances.

On the other hand, we can also find health benefits in using basti, and this can be another reason for taking it up along with any other shatkarmas that aid our health. Everyone is different and has different needs. However, obsession is never the right reason to undertake yoga practices, and especially not to overdo in them.

Obviously, we don't want to become dependent on basti for our elimination forever. If it is used mainly for health purposes, then maybe once or twice per week will be plenty. When the inner energies are moving (kundalini), our rising bhakti will let us know when it is time to do more basti and other shatkarmas. At times, it can be daily, and then, later on, maybe not at all.

In this discussion, we presented basti primarily as a spiritual practice. It is also utilized by many for health reasons. We have discussed a basic form of basti, which can be done by anyone at home. For health applications there are variations that may include more extensive assisted enemas in a clinical environment, and herbal enemas that contain various preparations added either to the enema water, or taken orally at a previous time. There are many variations available for using basti/enema.

For our purposes, a stable routine of practice will be the most effective approach during the time period on our path (weeks or months) that basti is needed.

Intestinal Wash

A more thorough and taxing method for cleansing the entire gastrointestinal (GI) tract is *dhauti*, or the *intestinal wash*, which entails drinking a large quantity of salted water. The salt prevents immediate digestion, and the water passes through the entire digestive tract, flushing everything in the digestive system out with it.

This procedure has been used by yoga practitioners for many centuries, and something similar to it is used in modern times to evacuate the digestive tract before a major medical procedure such as surgery.

Dhauti should not be done often. It depletes the system of natural biochemicals much more than basti does. Weekly would be considered to be very often for dhauti, and even monthly is often for this procedure. Several times per year, at most, is a more balanced approach to its use.

To perform dhauti, we drink two quarts or liters of salted water (two teaspoons of salt per quart or liter) slowly but steadily glass by glass over about fifteen minutes. Doing some light nauli (see below) between glasses of water is okay to aid in the inner flow. Then lie down on the left side (for best flow through intestines) for 20 minutes. Then go to the toilet, if the urge has not sent you there already.

It is best to plan on at least 30 minutes of eliminating off and on, and then lie down and rest afterward. The salt causes the water to pass straight through the entire GI tract for a big flush out. Besides the cleansing, this procedure can be temporarily depleting, due to the loss of biochemicals and vital essences in the GI tract.

In truth, basti (enema) is a more practical method. It can be done much more easily and quickly on a daily basis, if desired that often, and is not depleting. In fact, basti will increase the flow of inner energy, once ecstatic conductivity begins to arise in the neurobiology. Basti stimulates higher digestion in the GI tract, upstream from the colon, whereas dhauti temporarily suspends all digestion until the GI tract recovers from being completely flushed out. This is why it is recommended to use dhauti sparingly, particularly when ecstatic conductivity is on the rise.

More Shatkarmas

There are six traditional shatkarmas. There are many more, as many as the inner impulses of yoga can conjure up, including numerous variations on the shatkarmas being covered here. The six are *jala neti* (nasal wash), *basti* (colon cleansing/enema), *dhauti* (intestinal wash), *nauli* (churning of the abdominal muscles), *kapalbhati* (sudden exhale, a nerve cleansing pranayama method), and *trataka* (an eye/attention gazing method).

The first three of these shatkarmas are cleansing techniques in the physical sense, and have been covered. The remaining three are also physical, but do not involve flushing out the cavities of the body with water. They are more intimately involved in our daily yoga practices, and have, in fact, been covered to one degree or another in the AYP writings. If they have not been covered in name, then certainly in principle as applied in other practices in the overall routine of practices, including asanas, spinal breathing pranayama and deep meditation.

We will review these interconnections here.

Nauli

Nauli means *to churn*. It is a dynamic version of *uddiyana bandha* (abdominal lock), and consists of *twirling the abdominal muscles*, first in one direction, and then the other. Nauli stimulates the higher functioning of the digestive system by raising ecstatic kundalini energy up from the pelvic region into active participation with food and air in the GI tract, leading to whole body ecstatic conductivity. In the process, it provides stimulation for deep cleansing in the bowels. It can be practiced as part of asanas (yoga postures), and also during basti (enema) and dhauti (intestinal wash) to enhance cleansing and elimination when the bowels are full with saline water.

Before undertaking nauli, it is necessary to become proficient in uddiyana bandha, which is part of the routine of asanas undertaken before spinal breathing pranayama and deep meditation. For details on the asana routine, see the AYP book, *Asanas, Mudras and Bandhas*. In practicing uddiyana, we stand with feet shoulder-width apart with hands resting on knees. Then we expel the air fully from our lungs and pull the abdomen inward by lifting the diaphragm upward into the lung cavity. This is held for several five-second durations, or longer, as comfortable. Uddiyana means *to fly up*, which becomes apparent to many as soon as the practice is used. The inner energy literally flies up.

Nauli is a dynamic, or expanded, version of uddiyana, meaning it involves rhythmic movement, of the abdominal muscles, rather than holding a static position. The *churning* in nauli is accomplished by alternately flexing the left and right abdominal muscles to achieve a twirling effect. This is done in the same position as standing uddiyana, with air expelled and diaphragm lifted, while flexing the abdominal muscles (like when doing a sit-up), first against one knee through the supporting arm, and then against the other knee through the other supporting arm. This leads to the ability to control the flexing of left and right abdominal muscles separately, the key to accomplishing the twirling effect. Then nauli can be practiced any time in any position. It also becomes a less externally visible internal practice. It is a great aid to digestion and elimination.

Nauli is typically practiced during asanas at the same spot in the routine as uddiyana bandha, adding 10-20 twirls in each direction. Over time, nauli becomes a subtle automatic reflex in the body that contributes to vast inner flows of ecstatic energy. By then, cleansing has become very refined.

Further detailed instructions on uddiyana bandha and nauli can be found in the *AYP Easy Lessons for Ecstatic Living* book. Nauli is a powerful yoga practice and is best undertaken after the routine of asanas and sitting practices is well established. And then it should be measured and self-paced with prudence for steady, safe progress in its effects. A short duration of nauli practice will go a long way.

Kapalbhati

Kapalbhati means *shining forehead*. It is also interpreted to mean *luminous face*. It is a pranayama (breathing) technique, which involves taking a series of relaxed normal inhalations followed by sudden bellows-like exhalations. Inhalation is normally done through the nose, but can be done through the mouth if there is nasal obstruction. Exhalation is normally done through the nose also, but can also be done through the mouth with pursed lips to slightly restrict the exit of air. A primary effect of kapalbhati is to increase air pressure in short bursts in the nasal pharynx and sinuses, which stimulates the forward part of the brain. This provides a *brain cleansing*.

Kapalbhati can be repeated for a series of 10-20 cycles of relaxed inhalation and sudden exhalation. Be careful not to overdo this practice. A good time to practice kapalbhati is after yoga asanas and right before twice-daily sitting practices, which includes spinal breathing pranayama and deep meditation.

The effect of kapalbhati is purification of the neurobiology in the upper body, and in the head in particular. Hence the phrases, *shining forehead* and *luminous face*. It can give the internal sensation of energy radiating, and sometimes the external appearance of radiance in the face.

The principles and effects of kapalbhati are also found in spinal bastrika pranayama, which is a more advanced and broad-based practice utilized in daily sitting practices in the AYP system. Spinal bastrika also provides additional benefits for purification of the entire spinal nerve (sushumna) extending between the root (anus/perineum) and the center brow, and the entire nervous system radiating out from that central channel in us. Spinal bastrika pranayama may be selected over basic kapalbhati in daily sitting practices as our yoga routine advances over time.

Detailed instructions for spinal bastrika pranayama can be found in the *AYP Easy Lessons for Ecstatic Living* book.

Trataka

Trataka means *steady gazing*. It involves fixing the gaze on an object and leaving it there for a period of time. It purifies the inner machinery of attention, which in most of us comes out through the eyes for most of our waking hours. Fixing the gaze helps to loosen the grip of external experiences on the attention.

In many traditions, trataka, or some form of it, is used as a preparation for sitting practices. In some systems of practice, it is used as a primary meditation technique – the legendary practices of *candle gazing*, or *staring at a wall*.

In the AYP system of practices, we do not stare at a candle or a wall, at least not as a primary practice. Instead, we gently train the attention in inward ways to attend to the two primary processes of spiritual transformation that occur naturally in the human nervous system.

- The cultivation of *inner silence*, which is consciousness itself, before it has been focused as attention on any object. This is accomplished through deep meditation, and additional methods.

- The cultivation of *ecstatic conductivity*, which is the dynamic energetic aspect of our nature. This is accomplished with spinal breathing pranayama, and additional methods.

Both spinal breathing pranayama and deep meditation involve the use of attention – more sophisticated forms of steady gazing, we could say. In each case the primary technique is easy favoring a procedure utilizing attention *with eyes closed*, similar to how we would favor the object of our gazing with eyes open in trataka. Each time we wander off, we just easily bring the attention back. We are doing this with the simple procedures of spinal breathing pranayama and deep meditation. For the predetermined times of practice, they become our object of gazing, so to speak.

It might seem like a stretch to say that spinal breathing pranayama and deep meditation are forms of trataka. In fact, they are expansions on the principle, much in the way that spinal bastrika pranayama is an expansion on the principle of kapalbhati. It is taking basic principles and incorporating them into broader methods of practices, which are simple, yet far more global in their effects.

In AYP we use a simple form of trataka to aid in the development of *sambhavi mudra* during our spinal breathing pranayama, where the physical position of the eyes is separated from the movement of attention up and down the spinal nerve during inhalation and exhalation. In sambhavi, the eyes are raised and centered slightly, with an imperceptible furrowing of the center brow. This raising and centering of the eyes while they are closed is done during spinal breathing, while the attention is favoring cycling up and down the spinal nerve (center of the spinal column) between root and brow during inhalation and exhalation.

It takes some practice to learn to maintain sambhavi during spinal breathing, and a simple trataka exercise can help with this. It is done by keeping the eyes open and keeping a steady gaze on an external object while tracing the spinal nerve with the attention while breathing easily. This is neither spinal breathing pranayama, nor sambhavi mudra, but a preparation for doing sambhavi during spinal breathing. A little trataka like that will go a long way toward stabilizing our inner sambhavi practice (eyes closed) while we are doing spinal breathing pranayama, and a range of other yoga practices.

So, trataka can be a preparation for other practices by revealing to us the relationship of attention and the positioning of our eyes, and helping us develop better versatility with our attention in relation to the full range of practices we are doing. The principle of trataka (the favoring of an object or yoga procedure with attention) can be found in many practices.

As we have seen, the last three shatkarmas, or their underlying principles, are largely incorporated in the AYP system of practices already. Some additional benefits may be gained by practicing them separately in the traditional way. However, this may not be the ideal utilization of shatkarmas. The inner principles they stimulate through external manipulations are akin to the mudras and bandhas, and these kinds of practices are most effective when integrated with the core practices of spinal breathing pranayama and deep meditation. By *integrated*, we do not mean practiced at the same time. We mean combined in the daily routine in a way that optimizes the *effects* of our overall practice routine, which will facilitate steady progress in spiritual unfoldment with comfort and safety. Without comfort and safety, progress cannot be sustained, and sooner or later we will be compelled to curtail practices for a time. So, a wise course of action with practices is to engage in *self-pacing*, which means regulating practices in a way so as to balance progress with comfort and safety. At times this may mean not doing certain practices at all.

Shatkarmas are especially helpful if one is well-established in a steady routine of sitting practices, because there is a substantial spiritual dimension to them. Shatkarmas are an important aid for cultivating ecstatic conductivity in the neurobiology. The GI tract plays a central role in this, but not necessarily in the beginning days of our practices. It is much more important to become stable in our core practices.

From the AYP point of view, shatkarmas are middle stage practices, not needed much by most practitioners to enhance spiritual progress at the beginning or at the end of the journey. They are very helpful in the middle when ecstatic conductivity is coming into play. Of course, for health reasons, shatkarmas can be useful anytime, so they straddle the spiritual and physical health arenas, as do all yoga practices. Here we are focusing primarily on the spiritual side.

If we are involved in the AYP integrated application of deep meditation, spinal breathing pranayama, asanas, mudras and bandhas, we will have the principles of nauli, kapalbhati and trataka already incorporated into our daily routine. What will be new here is the *inner washing shatkarmas* – jala neti, basti and dhauti. In the case of these three, it is suggested to see how the rise of ecstatic conductivity stimulates our desire to do them, rather than forcing them prematurely into our daily routine. If we take this approach, a time for the inner washing shatkarmas will become clear. As the inner neurobiology begins to stir in the nasal passages, sinuses and GI tract, we will know when it is time to be providing extra cleansing in these areas. Ecstatic conductivity is cultivated mainly by spinal breathing pranayama, mudras, bandhas and additional forms of pranayama. Prerequisite to this is the rise of inner silence, which is cultivated mainly in deep meditation and samyama. So you can see there is a lot that will be happening before certain shatkarmas will be capable of producing their maximum effects.

This is the most practical way to approach the inner washing shatkarmas – when we feel called to them from within, then we do them. If not, then we will not be shortchanging ourselves spiritually by not doing them. Deep meditation, spinal breathing pranayama and other sitting practices are more important factors in our spiritual transformation. The *interconnectedness of yoga* will naturally call us to shatkarmas and the other yamas (restraints) and niyamas (observances) as our inner unfoldment requires. All yogic methods are part of the overall process of human spiritual transformation that resides within each of us.

Chapter 4 – Amaroli – Inner Rejuvenation

Amaroli means *urine therapy.* Since ancient times, in both the East and the West, urine therapy has been used to aid in curing many diseases. This has been accomplished by ingestion (the drinking of fresh urine – the primary form of amaroli), and also by applying fresh urine directly to wounds, sores, rashes and other visible maladies of the body. It has been claimed by enthusiastic adherents that urine therapy is capable of curing everything from asthma, the common cold and cancer – to hair loss, obesity and venereal disease. It will be left to the reader to research these claims. Much has been studied and recorded about urine therapy in relation to restoring and maintaining good health.

Urine therapy has also been used throughout the ages as a spiritual practice. In this book we are focused primarily on the role of urine therapy in yoga for promoting the process of human spiritual transformation. In the ancient and widely known *Hatha Yoga Pradipika*, the practice of urine therapy is called *Amaroli.* In the much more ancient and not as well known *Damar Tantra*, the practice is called *Shivambu Kalpa.* In both of these venerable scriptures, urine therapy is presented as an important spiritual practice.

So, if we are interested in maintaining good health and supplementing our yoga practice routine with an additional method that can help speed us along our way toward abiding inner silence, ecstatic bliss and outpouring divine love, then amaroli deserves a closer look.

Indeed, if we find the courage to try it, we may be pleasantly surprised. As they say, "The proof of the pudding is in the eating."

In this case, it is in the drinking.

How to do Amaroli – Urine Therapy

Whether it is being considered for health, spiritual practice, or both, Amaroli represents a paradox.

On one hand, amaroli walks headlong into a negative stigma many may have about drinking their own urine, even though this practice has been around for thousands of years and been used with success in many cultures. Yet, in the so-called *sanitized* cultures of today, the aversion is common.

On the other hand, amaroli has been shown clinically to have a wide range of health benefits, and may be one of the most effective healing tonics of all time. So much so that the pharmaceutical companies are in some cases selling back to us in pill form what we can obtain at much higher quality for free in the privacy of our own bathroom.

The truth is that daily urine therapy is one of the best things any of us can do as a preventive measure to ward off disease, and heal faster if we are suffering from just about any malady. Why is this? While it is still not fully understood, it is generally agreed by researchers that urine therapy enhances the presence of hundreds (or possibly thousands) of vital elements and compounds in our body, and builds our immune system to a strength beyond what it would be otherwise. Though less understood, amaroli also has been shown to have a purifying and rejuvenating effect in the body. All of that is pretty impressive, and we have not even begun to assess the spiritual benefits yet. What about the spiritual benefits?

It is notable that amaroli comes to us from ancient sources, not primarily because of its medicinal value, but for its value as a spiritual practice. In the *Hatha Yoga Pradipika* and the much older *Damar Tantra,* the goal of amaroli practice includes cultivating physical wellbeing, but reaches far beyond it, all the way out into the realm of enlightenment. It is worth overcoming long-held prejudices to get at the truth of the matter. The risk in this is nil, so amaroli is heartily recommended.

When we get up the courage to try, we will be wise to start small and build up. Isn't that how it is with most things in life, including our yoga practices? A traditional daily dose of urine is considered to be a glass full, or 6-8 ounces (200-250 milliliters). But we can start with a few drops, mixed with some water in a glass, and work up from there. There is no rule that says it has to end up being a full glass. It could be much less. What is important is daily practice – that much more important than the quantity. Everyone will be a bit different in their need and approach, as in all yoga practices.

When we engage in amaroli practice, the guideline is to do it first thing in the morning, whenever that is for us. When collecting urine, catch it *midstream*, which means after it starts and before it ends. As with many things, the first time will be the most daunting, even mixed with water. It will not harm you. The aversion is entirely psychological. Try it and see how you feel afterward.

If it is done in the shower and/or right before doing your oral hygiene in the morning, there will not be a trace of any odor by the time you leave the bathroom. It is an acquired taste, and is soon not offensive to the practitioner. Within a few days, it becomes much easier. Very easy, once the psychological barrier is broken. It is one of the easiest of all the yoga practices, much easier than any of the shatkarmas, and much easier than the mudras and bandhas. It can be a relatively quick journey from a few diluted drops to several undiluted swallows. Before you know it, the glass will be filling up and disappearing back into you again. That's daily amaroli practice. There isn't much more to it than that – except time. The longer we are doing it as a daily practice, the more the benefits accumulate.

It is not necessary to be drinking a full glass of urine every morning. In fact, it could be undesirable at certain times, or for certain people. There are several factors that could vary the dose. One is the quantity available. Another is the quality. If we have been eating heavily seasoned, salted, or fatty foods, or taking prescription drugs, the urine may be strong. Amaroli is not prohibited in any of these cases. The quantity may be curtailed or diluted with water as needed.

It is not recommended to mix urine with food or drink other than water, as this can reduce its effectiveness. The ideal time to do amaroli is on an empty stomach, with morning being best. We should wait at least fifteen minutes before eating after amaroli.

When the mouth is still wet with urine during amaroli, before drinking any water, several deep inhalations of the aromatic essence in the mouth will produce a soothing and healing influence in the lungs. Keep in mind that amniotic fluid in the womb is composed mainly of urine, and this is how we began our life before birth, doing amaroli, including in our lungs. So, inhaling some aromatic essence will not be harmful. Just the opposite – it is very beneficial for the lungs.

The practice of *self-pacing* is part of amaroli. If we are doing too much amaroli, we can have symptoms similar to those experienced when we do too much of any yoga practice – too many impurities coming out of the nervous system at once due to excessive purification going on inside.

If we are feeling any discomfort related to amaroli, then we know we should back off until things smooth out. We don't do practices at a level that makes us feel uncomfortable. Amaroli is no different than other yoga practices in this respect. So, if a full glass is proving to be too much, then try half a glass. If that is too much, start measuring swallows, and zero in on the right dose for yourself. It may be very little for some people, and more for others. Everyone is different. You won't find out what it is for you until you get into it.

In all of yoga, finding a balance between practices and our daily activities is an important part of the process. Once we have been on the path of yoga for a while, the right inner guidance always comes. Be flexible in that regard.

Enhancing the Subtle Biology for Inner Silence

Once we have been doing amaroli for a few weeks, we may notice something happening. Somehow we feel stronger inside – like some weak spaces deep inside us have been filled in. *Inwardly robust* is a phrase that comes to mind. We may not have noticed the weak spaces inside before, but we can feel that something has been filled in. That we will feel healthier goes without saying. Yes, definitely healthier. But there is something more, something beyond the feeling of the stronger, more stable physical presence that comes with daily amaroli practice. We can feel our awareness becoming more stable also.

One way to understand it is to think of our body and nervous system as the vehicle of our consciousness. When we strengthen the quality of our body and nervous system on the subtlest level of physicality, on the cellular level, we come to find ourselves living in a stronger and more reliable vehicle for our consciousness, our sense of self. This has a direct effect on our ability to maintain abiding inner silence.

When we sit to do practices, this gradual change in us that is being brought about by amaroli is noticeable also. The quality of our inner silence in meditation deepens and expands. The ecstatic energies we cultivate in spinal breathing pranayama and related practices, become more lively and luminous. The whole thing goes up a few notches with amaroli added into the daily schedule. And it keeps getting better over time, you know. As with the rest of our yoga, the effects of amaroli are cumulative, going ever deeper experientially over the months and years of our daily practice.

What is it that sets the condition for enlightenment in the human being? We have often said that it is a fundamental change in the condition of our nervous system, and the overall neurobiological functioning inside us. In other words, a primary prerequisite for enlightenment is raising the inner functioning of the human body to a much higher level. Then our vehicle of consciousness becomes capable of extraordinary expressions of the divine possibilities that are inherent within us. Bringing this change about is the purpose of yoga. We work systematically with our mind, our body, our emotions, our breath, and our sexuality to accomplish this transformation.

With amaroli, we are enhancing the chemical composition of our body at the most refined level, right down to the atoms and molecules. This creates a physiological foundation, adding an advantage as we engage in all of our other yoga practices that are propelling us along the road to enlightenment. That is the role of amaroli. We enjoy the benefits of our yoga practices in daily living every step along the way. This is why we engage in yoga practices, not necessarily for the experience while doing practices, but for the results we gain in daily living.

Amaroli is an important aspect of yoga. But it is not all of yoga. Its effects are greatly enhanced when combined with a daily routine including deep meditation, spinal breathing pranayama and other yoga methods. Likewise, amaroli improves the effectiveness of the other yoga practices. It is a balanced integration of practices that brings the

greatest enhancement in all aspects of li
mental, emotional and spiritual.

There is a tendency we all have
magic bullet, i.e., the one thing that
believe) will solve all things. Some
deep into one thing looking for that, only to
that they missed out on what a broader approach to self-improvement and spiritual development can yield. This is not to say that those who are strongly attracted to amaroli are wrong to pursue the practice with devotion. It is only to say that there are other practices to consider which can enhance our overall results when applied in a well-integrated daily routine.

Additional Aspects of Amaroli

We all have a tendency to think about individual spiritual practices in terms of their unique characteristics and effects. Amaroli is no exception in this, particularly since it is done at a time removed from our daily yoga postures and sitting practices. The truth is, amaroli can have a profound effect on our overall spiritual practices by virtue of the inner strength and integration it cultivates in the subtle realms of our physical body. Amaroli can also have additional positive effects in relation to other practices and the associated inner dynamics, as well as in preventive and curative healthcare.

Here we will take a look at four areas of interrelationship where urine therapy can play a significant role – in fasting, in healing compresses, in nasal wash, and in natural vajroli (rising sexual energy).

Amaroli with Fasting

As we have discussed in Chapter 2, occasional moderate fasting can be a useful practice which will bring inner cleansing and healing as our body takes a break from digestion and naturally applies its full

...gy to our inner purification. When amaroli is ...ded to a period of fasting, the cleansing and purification effects can be greatly amplified.

How much amaroli? And how much fasting?

Well, it is not recommended to begin both of these practices for the first time at the same time. Better to be established in one of them with good stability and results before adding the other.

For example, say we have been doing a monthly 24 hour fast, and feel we are ready to take on more purification during our fast. Of course, we could try increasing our fasting time to 48 hours. That would be one approach. Another approach could be to add amaroli. If we have already been practicing amaroli during our regular daily routine, we can try increasing amaroli practice from once per day to twice, or even three times per day during a fast. Of course, we would continue to take fluids as a normal part of our fast to maintain good hydration. Besides through urination, the body expels water through the respiratory system, perspiration, and the GI tract.

Whatever our choices may be for fasting with amaroli included, we should self-pace our practice (scale back as needed) if there is excessive discomfort. There is only so much purification we can assimilate over any given time period, so we pace things accordingly for good progress with comfort and safety.

In the case of serious illnesses, remarkable healing results can be achieved from fasting with amaroli, particularly if longer fasts and larger doses of amaroli are undertaken. However, in the case of a serious illness, it is recommended that, beyond the conservative approach described here, amaroli with fasting be applied with the assistance of an experienced therapist, and with the consultation of a medical doctor.

Urine Compresses for Wounds and Skin Ailments

The application of urine externally for helping to cure wounds and skin ailments is an ancient practice. While not very much in use in modern times, it is still practiced by those to whom the ancient knowledge has been passed down, and who are well aware of its benefits. External use of urine is most effective in combination with basic amaroli (urine ingestion), which provides the broadest coverage in the body. If daily amaroli is being practiced, external application may be considered to be a supplemental method.

Urine can be massaged into an afflicted area and then a urine-soaked compress can be applied. Only fresh urine should be used, preferably from the patient, and compresses should be changed every eight hours, or more often if practical.

Many will have an aversion to the external use of urine. As with amaroli itself, the benefits of external application of urine will likely be found to outweigh the concerns. A stigma cannot stand for long in the face of good results. Each can make their own decision about the benefits.

When urine compresses are added, as needed, during an amaroli fast, the maximum healing effect will be achieved. When considering any natural healing method, a medical doctor should be consulted to make sure all options, both ancient and modern, have been taken into account.

Of course, external application of urine for wounds and skin ailments does not have much bearing on our spiritual progress, except as maintaining good health does. That is a good enough reason to consider it. We need our health to be actively engaged in yoga practices.

Using Urine with Nasal Wash

Using urine with nasal wash is called *mutra neti*, rather than *jala neti*, and it is an age-old practice. Even so, it is an unconventional practice whose drawbacks may exceed its benefits much of the time. It is not recommended as a daily practice, except for short durations when the inner call for it is strong, or possibly in cases where there is a marked need for cleansing and healing in the nasal passages and/or sinuses. If there is a medical condition, a doctor's advice should be obtained so the option for the benefits of modern medicine will also be there for the treatment of any serious condition.

As with jala neti, salt content is the main determinant of comfort in mutra neti. Too much salt, like in seawater or most undiluted urine, can cause discomfort. Diluting the urine with water will reduce the salt content if this is necessary. It can be a tricky business, because the salt content of urine will vary from day to day. If we wish to practice mutra neti, but are deterred by the concentration or odor, just a few drops in our neti solution will be a good place to start. Some additional salt may be required to find the right balance for comfort. Once we become familiar with the practice, the urine content can be increased with less salt added, like that. Everyone has their own ideal salt level that is comfortable in the delicate nasal passages and sinuses.

The rest of the nasal wash procedure is the same as described in the last chapter. Add urine, or not, to suit the current need. Most will prefer not, and that is understandable. Only a few will want to try this. Our enlightenment does not depend on it.

The most important utilization of amaroli is in daily morning ingestion, which is an easy and comfortable practice to do once the habit has been established, and the positive results are readily observable in most people. Likewise, doing jala neti (nasal wash) with ordinary salted water on a daily basis during times of need, according to our intuition, will provide the lion's share of the benefits from this practice.

We do yoga practices for the positive results they bring with the greatest efficiency.

Amaroli and Natural Vajroli

Vajroli is a practice described in the *Hatha Yoga Pradipika*, and involves the drawing up of sexual fluids inside the body. In the AYP system of practices we do not go to the extremes that are described in this ancient treatise on yoga. Rather, natural vajroli is achieved through a full range of yoga practices, including deep meditation, spinal breathing pranayama, asanas, mudras, bandhas, tantric sexual techniques, and other methods.

By *natural vajroli*, we mean a natural drawing up of sexual essences through the urethra into the bladder and through many pathways upward in the neurobiology. This natural upward migration of vital essences gradually evolves to become a full-time occurrence in the life of the spiritual practitioner. This process occurs in both men and women, and is an integral part of the rise of full-time ecstatic conductivity in the body, which evolves further to become ecstatic radiance going out beyond the body.

In conjunction with this evolution in the sexual neurobiology, it may be observed that there is a gradual internalization of amaroli to become an automatic recycling within, which can result in less outflow. While there is no scientific verification of the internal recirculation of urine via natural vajroli, it has been observed in enough cases to be worthy of mention. It is well known that urination can become quite irregular with the awakening and advancement of kundalini (ecstatic conductivity). Whether amaroli itself plays a role in this evolution is not known. It will suffice to say that there is a relationship between amaroli and vajroli. This is pointed to in the *Hatha Yoga Pradipika*, and has been observed in practitioners in modern times, as well.

The integrated application of a full range of yoga practices gives rise to this phenomenon. It is also related to long term engagement in yoga practices. The changes described do not occur overnight, which is why a steady daily routine of practices that can be sustained long term is advised.

The extreme elements of practice which are sometimes seized upon by enthusiastic aspirants do not make a great difference in the overall scheme of things, because they cannot be sustained over the long term. Nor should they be. It is the practices we can engage in easily in a balanced way as part of our normal daily routine that will carry us steadily forward to the rising condition of abiding inner silence, ecstatic bliss and outpouring divine love.

We will know it is working for us as we find the practical results of the transformation emerging from within us day by day in our daily activities.

Chapter 5 – Putting It All Together

There is much that can be pondered when considering yogic diet, cleansing methods, and amaroli. On the other hand, with a sound foundation of inner silence, cultivated in daily deep meditation, everything will naturally find its appropriate role in our overall routine. This is assuming we do not go off the deep end with any particular practice. More and more of any yoga practice is not necessarily going to lead to the desired results. A well-balanced routine is by far the better approach.

This is why we have said at the beginning, "All things in moderation…"

While diet and cleansing methods are less esoteric than most of the practices covered in the AYP writings, meaning they can be learned in many places, there is a hidden pitfall in these methods. Because dietary and hygienic methods are intimately intertwined with our lifestyle, they can sometimes become obsessive behaviors, which will be counter-productive to our spiritual progress. It is the *magic bullet* mentality and *flights of fancy* that beckon us to the belief that one solution fits everyone at all times. Obviously, this is not so.

So the recommendation here is to integrate methods in a balanced way, as we are called to from within. While this may seem like an abstract approach, it really will not be if we are steady in our daily sitting practices over the long term. With that, we will naturally gravitate toward a lighter, more nutritious diet, and the cleansing and rejuvenation methods that are appropriate for the spiritual purification and opening that is occurring within us at any point in time. This is a natural integration of the methods described in this book in a way that will not be an imposition on our lifestyle and rising joy in everyday living. Indeed, the integration of lifestyle choices, including our diet and hygienic activities, are part of our rising inner joy, hastening its unfoldment.

This is how the methods in this book can be put together most effectively, through daily sitting practices and a balanced combination of our rising inner intuition and the application of good common sense. As is always the case in the AYP approach to spiritual practices, we take things one step at a time, always being mindful of causes and effects, and making adjustments as necessary for stable growth with comfort and safety.

There is no correct order by which diet and cleansing methods are to be taken on. If we have been meditating for a few months, we may be called to a lighter more nutritious diet, to shatkarmas, or perhaps to amaroli. We may be called to all of these at once, which is where our common sense comes in – taking things one step at a time to avoid overdoing. Rome was not built in a day.

Or we may not be called to any of these means. That is okay. If we are engaged in daily sitting practices, our inner purification and opening will be happening, and all will follow from that.

The Ecstatic Body

Because the methods in this book are associated primarily with the body, the approaches to diet, shatkarmas and amaroli described here are mainly concerned with enhancing the neurobiology of our inner ecstatic energy flow.

On the other side of the equation is the cultivation of inner silence, which is accomplished primarily through deep meditation and samyama.

While there is no doubt that inner silence is the source of our intuition (inner call) to engage in more methods of purification, it is also true that the application of yogic diet, shatkarmas and amaroli will enhance the rise of inner silence. But not very much without daily deep meditation in the picture. It is the effective integration of practices that makes the difference.

Before we may be called from within to change our diet, or engage in cleansing methods or amaroli, we will have the opportunity to include spinal breathing pranayama, asanas, mudras, bandhas, and tantric sexual techniques in our practices. These are all concerned with stimulating the rise of ecstatic conductivity and radiance in the body (kundalini). Once we have the beginnings of an *ecstatic body*, the role of diet, shatkarmas and amaroli will likely become obvious to us, and we will act accordingly.

The experience of rising inner ecstasy is multi-faceted and highly complex, enlivening every cell within us simultaneously. Yet, there is a central dynamic occurring in the ecstatic body, which is easily observed and interacted with. This is the awakening of the central spinal nerve (sushumna), and the rise of a luminous biochemistry in the gastrointestinal (GI) tract.

As our spinal nerve begins to open ecstatically, it will be very noticeable when we raise our eyes slightly toward the point between the eyebrows (sambhavi mudra), raise our tongue to the roof of our mouth or above the soft palate (kechari mudra), lightly squeeze our anus and perineum (mulabandha/asvini), gently lift our diaphragm (uddiyana/nauli), and naturally suspend our breath (kumbhaka). Any or all of these subtle activities will send ecstatic energy coursing through our body, and beyond. The flowing energies themselves also stimulate the performance of these activities by natural reflex. All aspects of yoga are connected internally in this way.

The digestive function is intimately interwoven in this process, providing the refined essences that support the ecstatic body. Hence, at some point we will naturally be inclined toward at least some of the approaches and methods described in this book, to further facilitate the ecstatic neurobiology and flow in the body. It is a natural process of unfoldment, which leads ultimately to a full time condition of abiding inner silence, ecstatic bliss, and outpouring divine love.

Self-Pacing in Practices

In the old days, we could go to a teacher, or *guru*, and the teacher would tell us what practices to do. If something went out of balance with our practices, we'd go back to the teacher and he or she would tell us what adjustments to make, and so on, back and forth. If our teacher happened to be on the other side of town, or on the other side of the world, we might be out of luck. This led to most spiritual teaching being done only in certain places on earth and to small numbers of practitioners who were fortunate to be near those places. This is the story of the transmission of spiritual knowledge over many centuries. Not very efficient. So it stands to reason that spiritual practices have historically been available to very few people, or what we call *esoteric*.

Now that we are in the *information age*, knowledge can be quickly conveyed to practitioners everywhere. And quick feedback is available too via the internet. Has the new technology solved the challenge of prescribing adjustments in practices to accommodate ongoing changes in experiences? Only in part. While communications have greatly improved, and much more information on practices is available, adjustments in practices still require very close supervision. In fact, the adjustments require supervision closer than any teacher has *ever* been able to provide, whether it is an old time guru who may be close by, or any teacher we happen to be in touch with via the internet. Guidance from another simply isn't enough. It has never been enough. It must come from within us. The true guru is in us, and always has been.

Enhanced spiritual progress becomes possible for anyone as soon as this important fact has been grasped. One of the first manifestations of this self-sufficiency is the rise of prudent *self-pacing* with powerful spiritual practices, and dramatic and safe spiritual progress that has not been available to large numbers of people in the past.

Nowadays we are finding that nearly everyone has the ability to self-pace their practices to compensate for changes in experiences as inner purification undergoes its unique course of progress in each individual. All that is needed are some basic instructions on symptoms of excess and how to compensate for these in practices.

Self-pacing is not only the key to maintaining a stable routine of practices we are already doing. Self-pacing is also the key to taking on new practices. It is about maintaining stability in practices with what we are already doing, while maintaining stability as we add on new practices as well.

This knowledge applies to all sitting practices, and to every other aspect of practice we may introduce in our daily life, including changes in our diet or the addition of shatkarmas and amaroli.

The key to expanding our practices is to be stable in all that we are doing already, and then adding on in increments, seeing what the experience is, and then making adjustments as necessary to maintain stability in practices over time. If this is not done, we can find ourselves in a situation where we have piled on too much, and then the entire program is at risk of being terminated by necessity, due to excessive uncomfortable symptoms. Then we have no practice at all. Much better to build up gradually, step-by-step.

So, if we have been doing deep meditation for a few weeks or months, and feel the urge to eat a lighter diet (this is natural), the way to answer this urge is not necessarily to go all at once to a strict vegan diet (no animal products, including dairy). A strong desire could be there, but if we force our conduct in that direction too quickly, it will be difficult to sustain a lasting change with stability. More likely we would be forced to revert back to where we started to reduce the strain.

This is the problem with all extreme diet changes – they rarely stick. Or any radical change in lifestyle habit. They rarely last. Much better to go in steps that we can assimilate and live with over time, and gravitate gradually in the direction our inner voice is calling us. This is a key part of self-pacing. It is tempering our spiritual desire (bhakti) with common sense. Our spiritual desire can be quite overwhelming at times, calling us to extreme and unsustainable measures. Our common sense knows better. This is the power of self-pacing.

Our spiritual desire would like us to be enlightened today, but our body needs some time to accomplish the task. It can be done, by applying an effective integration of means, with prudent self-pacing over time.

Once we have made a change in our practices, diet, etc., there will be many times along the way when adjustments will be necessary. If we adjust our practices as necessary, we will be able to continue our progressive routine with stability over the long term. If we do not self-pace, we will run into difficulties that can compromise our overall journey.

No one else can do self-pacing for us. Once we have the principles in hand, it is up to us to use them wisely. It is especially important when considering diet changes, shatkarmas or amaroli, which represent new introductions into our daily lifestyle, rather than adjustments in our routine of sitting yoga practices, which are more easily quantified. We will know it is time for adjustments if we are called to them from within. The inner call may be very strong. It is up to us to self-pace changes in our routine to assure long term spiritual progress with comfort and safety. It can be done!

Stillness in Action

There are several reasons why you may be reading this book. Maybe to help address some health concerns. Or maybe to explore diet, shatkarmas and amaroli as they relate to spiritual development.

Regardless of the reason we have been studying these things, we are all looking for the same thing – *Happiness*.

To some of us, happiness may mean *good health*. To others, happiness may mean *enlightenment*. We are all looking for it in our own way.

Fortunately, if we are pursuing a practical path of yoga practices, including the principles and methods discussed in this book, we will be improving both our health and our progress toward enlightenment. Our reasons are not nearly as important as our actions. When we have reasons that motivate us toward action, then those reasons, whatever they may be, are good enough. The reasons are a blessing, even if they might not seem so in the moment – like unhappiness in our personal life, or an adverse health situation. Either one will drive us to seek a solution. When we see an opening, a glimmer of light, we should move steadily toward it. When we seek, we will find. We will hear the inner call.

There is much to be gained by exploring and utilizing yoga methods, even just a little. Of course, steady practice over months and years will bring us many more benefits. Experiencing an unending inner happiness is possible if we are determined and keep up our practices over the long term. There will be many rewards along the way.

Progress in all of yoga is based on the cultivation of inner silence, which is accomplished through daily deep meditation. It is not difficult – only two short sittings per day and we will have all we need to be building a foundation of inner silence within us, which stimulates all other yoga practices, including the approaches to diet, shatkarmas and amaroli.

In the short run and in the long run it is about inner silence, or inner stillness. As we progress, stillness *moves* within us, and out from us to our external environment. This is how our behavior is uplifted in so many ways.

As we become still inside, we begin to move in ways that benefit us and those who are around us. We call this *stillness in action*.

It is not a featureless process. Stillness in action is filled with bliss and ecstasy. It is filled with love and purpose. Stillness in action is pure happiness.

What has this got to do with our diet and these cleansing techniques? What has it got to do with urine therapy?

Our body is the temple of the divine, the *City of God*. We are the doorway. To open our doorway to the divine flow that comes from within, there are many means that can be applied – deep meditation, spinal breathing pranayama, postures and inward physical maneuvers. Even our sexuality can be enlisted to promote our spiritual unfoldment.

While what we eat and the inner hygiene methods we perform may not be the primary means for opening the doorway, they are important supporting methods in the whole of yoga. They constitute the branch of yoga called *purity*. All of the limbs of yoga are connected – each one stimulating the others. Our sitting practices will stimulate diet, shatkarmas and amaroli, and vice versa.

It is a multidimensional journey of integrated methods and steps, each undertaken with moderation, and balanced for best effects through self-pacing.

In the end, the totality of our life experience becomes stillness in action, a continuous divine flow found to be coming through us, and in everyone and everything around us. It is a condition of Oneness, ever still and ever moving in eternal joy.

Appendix

Ayurveda Diet Guidelines

Ayurveda is the ancient Indian system of natural healthcare and healing. Ayurveda means *knowledge of life and longevity*. Unlike the modern western approach to healthcare, which is centered on treating disease when it arises, ayurveda is designed to first promote the prevention of disease through a balanced lifestyle, including daily yoga practices, and other measures that promote internal harmony and health. In cases where disease is present, ayurveda seeks the restoration of balance to facilitate the cure through self-healing. Even with all of its technology, modern medicine also relies on the healing powers within the patient. So, regardless of our approach to medicine, it will be the patient's natural healing processes we are always seeking to facilitate.

When things have gone so far out of balance that radical interventions with prescription drugs and/or surgery are necessary, then modern medicine can undoubtedly save lives, and we may find ourselves taking advantage of the benefits, and thankful for it. But at what cost?

Before it reaches the point where chronic disease has come over us, there is much that can be done with lifestyle and the gentle time-tested methods of ayurveda to cultivate our health and longevity. Therefore, we will be wise to take advantage of this ancient knowledge.

While there are many treatment modalities in ayurveda, including all the methods of yoga, we will only be looking at one of them in this appendix – the management of diet to aid in maintaining and restoring the balance of our inner energies. To learn more about the broad range of methods available in ayurveda, consult a qualified ayurvedic physician, clinic or self-study program.

Diet has a particular significance on the spiritual path, where the ongoing purification and opening of our neurobiology can place challenges on the balance of our inner energies. As discussed in Chapter 2, the digestive system plays a key role in this development, so we will take a closer look at diet from an ayurvedic point of view.

At the heart of ayurveda are the *doshas*, the three inner biological humors, which determine an individual's constitution: *Vata* (movement), *Pitta* (heat), and *Kapha* (structure). The therapies of ayurveda promote balance of the doshas, which provides a foundation for good physical and spiritual health. This is accomplished by *balancing* or *pacifying* one or more doshas that are too strong in relation to the others.

How will we know which of our doshas is out of balance?

The first consideration will be our inherent bodily constitution. This is what we were born with. We each have tendencies in us that determine how energy (prana) will flow through our body.

The second consideration will be any particular imbalance we may be experiencing in the present, which will be influenced by our inherent constitution, plus our lifestyle, including personal habits, diet, environment and the conduct of our spiritual practices.

We can develop a general idea about how the doshas are manifesting in us by observing the following:

- **Vata** – Movement of thoughts, emotions and body. <u>Is our nature active, flexible and inquiring</u>, or are we moving around so much that effective activity eludes us? Are mind and emotions racing?

- **Pitta** – The amount of heat generated in our body, particularly in digestion. <u>Is our nature focused and active</u>, or fiery and angry? Are we prone to skin rashes?

- **Kapha** – The degree of structure in our nature and life. <u>Is our nature steady and reliable</u>, or are we stuck in inertia? Do we have trouble getting up to do things? Are we prone to gain weight?

Detailed assessments of our doshas can be obtained from an ayurvedic physician and through the many self-evaluation programs available. We are each a mixture of the traits mentioned. When our doshas are in balance, we will experience more of the desirable dosha traits, which are underlined above. And if one or more of our doshas are out of balance, we may experience some of the undesirable symptoms.

The Six Tastes and Balancing the Doshas

Diet can play a key role in balancing the doshas. This is done through management of the intake of different types of foods, which are categorized by the six tastes and how they affect our inner constitution. The six tastes and the types of foods they are associated with include:

1. **Sweet** – Fruit, grains, sugars, milk.
2. **Sour** – Sour fruits, yogurt, fermented foods.
3. **Salty** – Natural and unnatural salts, sea vegetables.
4. **Bitter** – Dark leafy greens, certain herbs and spices.
5. **Pungent** (strong) – Chili peppers, garlic, certain herbs and spices.
6. **Astringent** (drying) – Legumes, raw fruits and vegetables, and certain herbs.

The six tastes are inclined to balance or aggravate the three doshas as shown in this table:

Taste	Vata	Pitta	Kapha
Sweet	Balance	Balance	Aggravate
Sour	Balance	Aggravate	Aggravate
Salty	Balance	Aggravate	Aggravate
Bitter	Aggravate	Balance	Balance
Pungent	Aggravate	Aggravate	Balance
Astringent	Aggravate	Balance	Balance

With this information, we can construct a complete ayurvedic diet to aid in balancing our inner energies, which will help maintain good health. Note that herbs and spices are mentioned in the taste categories above. They can play a significant role in balancing the doshas, as generally indicated in the food charts in this appendix. More targeted utilization of herbs, spices and other ayurvedic (mineral) supplements is an important field of knowledge for dealing with chronic dosha imbalances, and experts in this specialized field can be consulted as needed.

By reviewing the chart above, we can see how poor diet has been a contributing factor to health issues in our modern society. This is no secret. It is well known that a heavy focus on carbohydrates (sweet), fermented (sour), and salty foods has lead to an epidemic of health problems in many countries. It would not be such a problem if everyone were vata in their inherent constitution. But this is not the case. One diet does not fit all, and this is the primary message in these ayurveda diet guidelines.

Inwardly we know this, and this is why we are called to variations in diet as we advance in yoga practices.

Of particular significance in yoga is the awakening of our inner ecstatic energies (kundalini), which stimulate a wide range of neurobiological changes within us, and can lead to imbalances in our doshas. The signature dosha imbalance for kundalini is pitta – a lot of heat being generated in the body as the neurobiology is being purified by greatly increased inner energy flow. This is often accompanied by a vata imbalance (lots of inner energy movement), so it is not uncommon for there to sometimes be both a pitta and vata imbalance as we move ahead on our spiritual path into the awakening of ecstatic conductivity and radiance. Utilizing ayurvedic diet measures can help during these times, smoothing our journey along the road to enlightenment.

The charts on the following pages have been constructed utilizing the basic taste and dosha criteria discussed above. While the foods shown are primarily from the western hemisphere, the same criteria can be used to favor or avoid foods from anywhere according to their predominant taste characteristics. Using such a chart can be helpful when we are on our way to the food cupboard or refrigerator, assuming we know which of our doshas are out of balance. It is not hard to tell with some basic knowledge in hand.

None of these diet guidelines are iron-clad. For example, if you are having a classic kundalini imbalance involving both pitta and vata, then what to do? The vata and pitta balancing diets are at odds in some categories, but not in all. It becomes a matter of tiptoeing through the inner energies, favoring pitta balancing foods here, and vata balancing foods there, according to the experiences of the day, week and month. With some persistence and self-pacing in utilizing various types of foods, this approach can work. Getting the diet right is often a process of trial and error. So it is in dealing with any combination of dosha imbalances.

There is also the matter of incorporating the modern knowledge of balancing the consumption of carbohydrates, proteins and fats in moderation, while maintaining a healthy intake of fruits, vegetables, fiber and fluids. There are many factors to consider when mixing ancient and modern knowledge. If we are wise in our choices, we can benefit from the best of both worlds as we advance on our spiritual path. The ayurveda diet charts reveal many opportunities.

On the path of yoga, there can be shifts in dosha balances as the inner energies become active and are purifying the nervous system at rapid rate. Interestingly, as we continue our yoga practices through all of these changes, we eventually arrive at a state where we become largely impervious to the effects of just about any kind of food. This is true at least as diet relates to our spiritual condition, where we have become abiding inner silence, ecstatic bliss, and outpouring divine love. Our spiritual development eventually moves beyond the effects of food, or the state of our doshas. Then diet is much less critical in relation to the condition of our consciousness, though we may continue to eat a healthy diet for the sake of our physical health and longevity. Why not?

In the meantime, we can aid both our spiritual journey and our physical health with some attention on diet. The ayurvedic diet suggestions on the following charts can help when used with good common sense in conjunction with a daily routine of yoga practices – deep meditation, spinal breathing pranayama, etc. Yoga practices also aid in balancing our doshas, when applied prudently using the principles of self-pacing to best advantage.

The following three tables provide diet suggestions for balancing the doshas – *Vata, Pitta and Kapha*.

Eleven food categories are covered for each dosha, including: Fruits, Vegetables, Grains, Animal Foods, Legumes, Nuts, Seeds, Sweeteners, Condiments (seasonings), Dairy, and Oils.

Eat wisely for smooth spiritual progress, good health and longevity – and enjoy!

Vata Balancing Diet Suggestions

	Balancing?	Favor or Avoid
Fruits	Yes	Sweet fruits, apricots, avocado, bananas, berries, cherries, coconut, figs (fresh), grapefruit, grapes, lemon, mango, melons (sweet), oranges, papaya, peaches, pineapple, plums
	No	Dried fruits, apples, cranberries, pears, persimmon, pomegranate, watermelon
Vegetables	Yes	Cooked vegetables, asparagus, beets, carrots, cucumber, garlic, green beans, okra (cooked), onion (cooked), potatoes (sweet), radishes, zucchini
	No	Raw vegetables, broccoli, brussels sprouts, cabbage, cauliflower, celery, eggplant, leafy greens, lettuce*, mushrooms, onions (raw), parsley*, peas, peppers, potatoes (white), spinach*, sprouts*, tomatoes (* indicates Okay in moderation with oil dressing)
Grains	Yes	Oats (cooked), rice, wheat
	No	Barley, buckwheat, corn, millet, oats (dry), rye
Animal Foods	Yes	Beef, chicken/turkey (white meat), eggs (fried/scrambled), seafood
	No	Lamb, pork, rabbit, venison
Legumes	Yes	Mung beans, tofu, black & red lentils
	No	All other legumes
Nuts	Yes	All nuts in small quantities
Seeds	Yes	All seeds in moderation
Sweeteners	Yes	All sweeteners except white sugar
	No	White sugar
Condiments	Yes	All spices are good
Dairy	Yes	All dairy in moderation
Oil	Yes	All oils are good

Pitta Balancing Diet Suggestions

	Balancing?	Favor or Avoid
Fruits	Yes	Sweet fruits, apples, avocado, coconut, figs, grapes (dark), mango, melons, oranges (sweet), pears, pineapple (sweet), plums (sweet), pomegranate, prunes, raisins
	No	Sour fruits, apricots, berries, bananas, cherries, cranberries, grapefruit, grapes (green), lemons, oranges (sour), papaya, peaches, pineapples (sour), persimmon, plums (sour)
Vegetables	Yes	Sweet & bitter vegetables, asparagus, broccoli, brussels sprouts, cabbage, cucumber, cauliflower, celery, green beans, leafy greens, lettuce, mushrooms, okra, peas, parsley, peppers (green), potatoes, Sprouts, zucchini
	No	Pungent vegetables, beets, carrots, eggplant, garlic, onions, peppers (hot), radishes, spinach, tomatoes
Grains	Yes	Barley, oats (cooked), rice (basmati), rice (white), wheat
	No	Buckwheat, corn, millet, oats (dry), rice (brown), rye
Animal Foods	Yes	Chicken/turkey (white meat), eggs (whites), rabbit, shrimp (small amount), venison
	No	Beef, eggs (yoke), lamb, pork, seafood
Legumes	Yes	All legumes except lentils
	No	Lentils
Nuts	Yes	Coconut
	No	All other nuts
Seeds	Yes	Sunflower, pumpkin
	No	All other seeds
Sweeteners	Yes	All sweeteners except molasses and honey
	No	Molasses, honey
Condiments	Yes	Coriander, cinnamon, cardamom, fennel, turmeric, black pepper (small amount)
	No	All other spices
Dairy	Yes	Butter (unsalted), cottage cheese, ghee, milk
	No	Buttermilk, cheese, sour cream, yogurt
Oil	Yes	Coconut, olive, sunflower, soy
	No	Almond, corn, safflower, sesame

Kapha Balancing Diet Suggestions

	Balancing?	Favor or Avoid
Fruits	Yes	Apples, apricots, berries, cherries, cranberries, figs (dry), mango, peaches, pears, persimmon, pomegranate, prunes, raisins
	No	Sweet & sour fruits, avocado, bananas, coconut, figs (fresh) grapefruit, grapes, lemons, melons, oranges, papaya, pineapple, plums
Vegetables	Yes	Pungent & bitter vegetables, asparagus, beets, broccoli, brussels sprouts, cabbage, carrots, cauliflower, celery, eggplant, garlic, leafy greens, lettuce, mushrooms, okra, onions, parsley, peas, peppers, Potatoes (white), radishes, spinach, sprouts
	No	Sweet & juicy vegetables, cucumber, potatoes (sweet), tomatoes, zucchini
Grains	Yes	Barley, corn, millet, oats (dry), rice (small amount – basmati), rye
	No	Oats (cooked), rice (brown), rice (white), wheat
Animal Foods	Yes	Chicken/turkey (dark meat), eggs (not fried or scrambled), rabbit, shrimp, venison
	No	Beef, lamb, pork, seafood
Legumes	Yes	All legumes except as listed
	No	Kidney beans, soy beans, black lentils, mung beans
Nuts	No	No nuts at all
Seeds	Yes	Sunflower, pumpkin
	No	All other seeds
Sweeteners	Yes	Raw honey
	No	All other sweeteners
Condiments	Yes	All condiments except salt
	No	Salt
Dairy	Yes	Ghee, goat milk
	No	All other dairy
Oil	Yes	Almond, corn, sunflower (all in moderation)
	No	All other oils

Further Reading and Support

Yogani is an American spiritual scientist who, for more than thirty years, has been integrating ancient techniques from around the world which cultivate human spiritual transformation. The approach he has developed is non-sectarian, and open to all. In the order published, his books include:

Advanced Yoga Practices – Easy Lessons for Ecstatic Living
A large user-friendly textbook providing 240 detailed lessons on the AYP integrated system of yoga practices.

The Secrets of Wilder – A Novel
The story of young Americans discovering and utilizing actual secret practices leading to human spiritual transformation.

The AYP Enlightenment Series
Easy-to-read instruction books on yoga practices, including:

- *Deep Meditation – Pathway to Personal Freedom*
- *Spinal Breathing Pranayama – Journey to Inner Space*
- *Tantra – Discovering the Power of Pre-Orgasmic Sex*
- *Asanas, Mudras and Bandhas – Awakening Ecstatic Kundalini*
- *Samyama – Cultivating Stillness in Action, Siddhis and Miracles*
- *Diet, Shatkarmas and Amaroli – Yogic Nutrition and Cleansing for Health and Spirit*
- *Self Inquiry – Dawn of the Witness and the End of Suffering*
- *Bhakti and Karma Yoga – The Science of Devotion and Liberation Through Action* (2nd half 2007)
- *Eight Limbs of Yoga – The Structure and Pacing of Self-Directed Spiritual Practice* (2nd half 2007)

For up-to-date information on the writings of Yogani, and for the free *AYP Support Forums*, please visit:

www.advancedyogapractices.com

Lightning Source UK Ltd.
Milton Keynes UK
UKOW04f1129160314

228206UK00001B/4/A